Teen Health Series

Diabetes Information for Teens,
Third Edition

Diabetes Information for Teens,
Third Edition

Health Tips about Managing Diabetes and
Preventing Related Complications

Including Facts about Insulin, Glucose Control,
Diabetes-Related Health Concerns, Healthy Eating,
Physical Activity, and Learning to Live with Diabetes

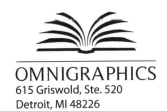

OMNIGRAPHICS
615 Griswold, Ste. 520
Detroit, MI 48226

Table of Contents

Preface

Part One: Understanding Diabetes

Chapter 1——Facts and Statistics about Diabetes...................................3

Chapter 2——Who Is at Risk for Diabetes? 9

Chapter 3——Diabetes in Children and Adolescents 13

Chapter 4——Metabolic Syndrome: An Early Warning Sign 17

Chapter 5——Insulin Resistance and Prediabetes.............................27

Chapter 6——Type 1 Diabetes 33

Chapter 7——Type 2 Diabetes 41

Chapter 8——Double Diabetes..47

Chapter 9——Gestational Diabetes and Diabetes-Related
           Women's Concerns 51

Chapter 10—Monogenic Forms of Diabetes 57

Chapter 11—Diabetes Myths 63

Part Two: Medical Management of Diabetes

Chapter 12—You and Your Diabetes Care Team 69

Chapter 13—Steps to Manage Your Diabetes for Life 75

Chapter 14—Know Your Blood Sugar Numbers 83

Chapter 15—Blood Glucose Monitoring...89

Chapter 16—Glucose in Urine Test...97

Chapter 17—Ketones in Urine Test 101

Chapter 18—Diabetes Medicines 105

Chapter 19—Insulin Delivery Devices... 111

Chapter 20—Managing Hypoglycemia... 115

Chapter 21—Managing Hyperglycemia.................................... 121

Chapter 22—Beware of Diabetes Treatment Fraud........................ 125

Part Three: The Physical Complications of Diabetes

Chapter 23—Diabetes-Related Health Concerns............................ 131

Chapter 24—Diabetes, Heart Disease, and Stroke.......................... 139

Chapter 25—Diabetic Neuropathy... 147

Chapter 26—Diabetic Eye Disease 153

Chapter 27—Diabetic Kidney Disease 161

Chapter 28—Gastroparesis.. 167

Chapter 29—Tooth and Gum Problems Caused by
                   Diabetes... 175

Chapter 30—Foot and Skin Problems Caused by
                   Diabetes... 183

Chapter 31—Acanthosis Nigricans and Necrobiosis
                   Lipoidica 191

Chapter 32—Sexual and Bladder Problems of Diabetes 193

Part Four: Mental Health and Lifestyle Issues

Chapter 33—The Link between Diabetes and
                   Mental Health 203

Chapter 34—Tips for Coping with Diabetes Distress...................... 207

Chapter 35—Diabetes Management at School............................. 211

Chapter 36—Importance of Wearing Medical Alert
                   Bracelets and Necklaces 215

Chapter 37—Driving When You Have Diabetes............................ 219

Chapter 38—Traveling When You Have Diabetes 223

Chapter 39—Take Care of Your Diabetes during
            Sick Days and Special Times 227

Chapter 40—Managing Diabetes in the Heat 235

Chapter 41—Smoking and Diabetes 239

Chapter 42—If Your Friend or Family Member Has
            Diabetes 243

Part Five: Nutrition, Physical Activity, and Weight Management

Chapter 43—Healthy Eating for Diabetics 249

Chapter 44—Making Healthy Food Choices 253

Chapter 45—Meal Plans and Diabetes 259

Chapter 46—Carbohydrate Counting 265

Chapter 47—Diabetes and Dietary Supplements 273

Chapter 48—Physical Activity and Diabetes 279

Chapter 49—Stay at a Healthy Weight... 285

Chapter 50—Early Weight-Loss Surgery May Improve
            Type 2 Diabetes and Blood Pressure
            Outcomes 289

Part Six: If You Need More Information

Chapter 51—Resources for Diabetes Information 295

Chapter 52—Finding Diabetes-Friendly Recipes 309

Index 327

Preface

About This Book

The teen years are especially important in the battle against diabetes. As young people begin to take more personal responsibility for managing their health, they make their own choices about what to eat and what activities to pursue. These decisions can have consequences that impact well-being throughout the adult years. Currently, efforts to overcome diabetes are making little progress. According to recent U.S. statistics, the prevalence of type 1 diabetes appears to be increasing among children and adolescents. Researchers suspect that a combination of genetic and environmental factors may be involved in a process that causes the body's autoimmune system to destroy insulin-producing pancreatic beta-cells. In addition, type 2 diabetes, which used to occur almost exclusively in adults, is now appearing with greater frequency among young people. Evidence suggests the trend is related to a tendency for children and adolescents to be more overweight and less active. However, medical advancements are helping people with diabetes better manage the disease, forestalling its complications. In addition, new insights into the disease's development are leading to more focused prevention efforts. In some cases, these involve lifestyle changes that can help delay—or even prevent—diabetes from developing. For people in whom the disease does appear, proper care and health management can help patients avoid its most serious long-term complications, such as nerve damage, loss of vision, amputation, kidney failure, and even premature death.

Diabetes Information for Teens, Third Edition examines the alarming trends in diabetes prevalence, and it provides information about positive steps that can be taken. The book provides facts about the different types of diabetes, its medical management, and the roles of nutrition and physical activity in averting its consequences. Suggestions are included for handling problematic situations, such as caring for diabetes at school or dealing with the emotional ups and downs associated with having diabetes, and a special section describes related health concerns and the prevention of complications. For readers seeking more information, the book provides a directory of diabetes resources and information about diabetes-friendly recipes.

How to Use This Book

This book is divided into parts and chapters. Parts focus on broad areas of interest; chapters are devoted to single topics within a part.

Part One: Understanding Diabetes begins with facts and statistics about diabetes. It explains how the metabolic processes that fuel the body can sometimes go awry leading to diabetes. It describes the differences between the many forms of diabetes, and myths about diabetes.

Part Two: Medical Management of Diabetes talks about the importance of working with a health-care team and self-monitoring blood glucose levels. It explains commonly used diabetes medications and discusses the different roles played by oral diabetes medications and insulin. Problems related to blood sugar levels that are too high or too low are addressed. It also sheds light on diabetes treatment frauds and unapproved diabetes drugs.

Part Three: The Physical Complications of Diabetes explains how the metabolic processes that lead to diabetes can also damage the heart, blood vessels, nerves, eyes, kidneys, and other organs and systems of the body. Suggestions for preventing—or at least delaying—these health consequences are also included.

Part Four: Mental Health and Lifestyle Issues looks at the emotional aspects of dealing with diabetes and how disease management practices interact with daily life. It explains how mental health is of special concern to people with diabetes, and it offers tips for dealing with diabetes in particular situations, such as at school, while driving and traveling, when sick, and so on.

Part Five: Nutrition, Physical Activity, and Weight Management includes facts about meal planning and dietary strategies that can help keep blood sugar levels within a target range. It also discusses the importance of physical activity as a disease-management tool, and it explains how achieving a healthy body weight can help keep diabetes better controlled.

Part Six: If You Need More Information offers a directory of resources for more information about diabetes and some interesting diabetes-friendly recipes.

Bibliographic Note

This volume contains documents and excerpts from publications issued by the following U.S. government agencies: Centers for Disease Control and Prevention (CDC); Genetic and Rare Diseases Information Center (GARD); National Center for Complementary and Integrative Health (NCCIH); National Heart, Lung, and Blood Institute (NHLBI); National Highway Traffic Safety Administration (NHTSA); National Institute of Diabetes and Digestive and Kidney Diseases (NIDDK); National Institutes of Health (NIH); U.S. Department of Veterans Affairs (VA); and U.S. Food and Drug Administration (FDA).

It may also contain original material produced by Omnigraphics and reviewed by medical consultants.

The photograph on the front cover is © Mark Hatfield/iStockphoto.

Medical Review

Omnigraphics contracts with a team of qualified, senior medical professionals who serve as medical consultants for the *Teen Health Series*. As necessary, medical consultants review reprinted and originally written material for currency and accuracy. Citations including the phrase "Reviewed (month, year)" indicate material reviewed by this team. Medical consultation services are provided to the *Teen Health Series* editors by:

Dr. Vijayalakshmi, MBBS, DGO, MD
Dr. Senthil Selvan, MBBS, DCH, MD
Dr. K. Sivanandham, MBBS, DCH, MS (Research), PhD

About the *Teen Health Series*

At the request of librarians serving today's young adults, the *Teen Health Series* was developed as a specially focused set of volumes within Omnigraphics' *Health Reference Series*. Each volume deals comprehensively with a topic selected according to the needs and interests of people in middle school and high school. Teens seeking preventive guidance, information about disease warning signs, medical statistics, and risk factors for health problems will find answers to their questions in the *Teen Health Series*. The Series, however, is not intended to serve as a tool for diagnosing illness, in prescribing treatments, or as a substitute for the physician/patient relationship. All people concerned about medical symptoms or the possibility of disease are encouraged to seek professional care from an appropriate healthcare provider.

If there is a topic you would like to see addressed in a future volume of the *Teen Health Series*, please write to:

Editor
Teen Health Series
Omnigraphics
615 Griswold, Ste. 520
Detroit, MI 48226

A Note About Spelling And Style

Teen Health Series editors use *Stedman's Medical Dictionary* as an authority for questions related to the spelling of medical terms and the *Chicago Manual of Style* for questions related to grammatical structures, punctuation, and other editorial concerns. Consistent adherence is not always possible, however, because the individual volumes within the Series include many documents from a wide variety of different producers and copyright holders, and the editor's primary goal is to present material from each source as accurately as is possible following the terms specified by each document's producer. This sometimes means that information in different chapters may follow other guidelines and alternate spelling authorities. For example, occasionally a copyright holder may require that eponymous terms be shown in possessive forms (Crohn's disease vs. Crohn disease) or that British spelling norms be retained (leukaemia vs. leukemia).

Part One
Understanding Diabetes

Chapter 1

Facts and Statistics about Diabetes

What Is Diabetes?

Diabetes is a disease that occurs when your blood glucose, also called "blood sugar," is too high. Blood glucose is your main source of energy and comes from the food you eat. Insulin, a hormone made by the pancreas, helps glucose from food get into your cells to be used for energy. Sometimes, your body does not make enough—or any—insulin, or it does not use insulin well. Glucose then stays in your blood and does not reach your cells.

Over time, having too much glucose in your blood can cause health problems. Although diabetes has no cure, you can take steps to manage your diabetes and stay healthy.

> Sometimes, people call diabetes "a touch of sugar" or "borderline diabetes." These terms suggest that someone does not really have diabetes or has a less serious case, but every case of diabetes is serious.

What Are the Different Types of Diabetes?

The most common types of diabetes are type 1, type 2, and gestational diabetes.

About This Chapter: Text beginning with the heading "What Is Diabetes?" is excerpted from "What Is Diabetes?" National Institute of Diabetes and Digestive and Kidney Diseases (NIDDK), November 2016; Text beginning with the heading "The Big Picture" is excerpted from "Diabetes Quick Facts," Centers for Disease Control and Prevention (CDC), May 11, 2018; Text beginning with the heading "Diabetes Incidence and Prevalence" is excerpted from "Diabetes Report Card 2017," Centers for Disease Control and Prevention (CDC), 2017.

Type 1 Diabetes

If you have type 1 diabetes, your body does not make insulin. Your immune system attacks and destroys the cells in your pancreas that make insulin. Type 1 diabetes is usually diagnosed in children and young adults, although it can appear at any age. People with type 1 diabetes need to take insulin every day to stay alive.

Type 2 Diabetes

If you have type 2 diabetes, your body does not make or use insulin well. You can develop type 2 diabetes at any age, even during childhood. However, this type of diabetes occurs most often in middle-aged and older people. Type 2 is the most common type of diabetes.

Gestational Diabetes

Gestational diabetes develops in some women when they are pregnant. Most of the time, this type of diabetes goes away after the baby is born. However, if you have had gestational diabetes, you have a greater chance of developing type 2 diabetes later in life. Sometimes, diabetes diagnosed during pregnancy is actually type 2 diabetes.

Other Types of Diabetes

Less common types include monogenic diabetes, which is an inherited form of diabetes, and cystic fibrosis-related diabetes.

How Common Is Diabetes?

As of 2015, 30.3 million people in the United States, or 9.4 percent of the population, had diabetes. More than 1 in 4 of them did not know they had the disease. Diabetes affects 1 in 4 people over the age of 65. About 90 to 95 percent of cases in adults are type 2 diabetes.

Who Is More Likely to Develop Type 2 Diabetes?

You are more likely to develop type 2 diabetes if you are 45 years of age or older, have a family history of diabetes, or are overweight. Physical inactivity; race; and certain health problems, such as high blood pressure, also affect your chance of developing type 2 diabetes. You are also more likely to develop type 2 diabetes if you have prediabetes or had gestational diabetes when you were pregnant.

The Big Picture

More than 30 million people in the United States have diabetes, and 1 in 4 of them do not know they have it.

- More than 84 million U.S. adults—over a third—have prediabetes, and 90 percent of them do not know they have it.

- Diabetes is the seventh leading cause of death in the United States (and may be underreported).

- Type 2 diabetes accounts for about 90 to 95 percent of all diagnosed cases of diabetes; type 1 diabetes accounts for about 5 percent.

- In the last 20 years, the number of adults diagnosed with diabetes has more than tripled as the American population has aged and become more overweight or obese.

Complications

People with diabetes are twice as likely to have heart disease or a stroke as people without diabetes—and at an earlier age.

- In the United States, diabetes is the leading cause of chronic kidney diseases, lower-limb amputations, and adult-onset blindness.

- Smokers are 30 to 40 percent more likely to develop type 2 diabetes than nonsmokers.

- People with diabetes who smoke are more likely to develop serious related health problems, including heart and kidney disease.

- In about 2 out of 3 American Indians/Alaska Natives with kidney failure, diabetes is the cause.

Cost

- Medical costs and lost work and wages for people with diagnosed diabetes total $327 billion yearly.

- Medical costs for people with diabetes are twice as high as for people who do not have diabetes.

Diabetes Incidence and Prevalence

Diabetes incidence—which is the rate of new cases of diagnosed diabetes—among adults in the United States went down in 2015 and has gone down each year since 2008 (Figure 1.1). About 1.4 million new cases of diabetes were diagnosed among adults between the ages of 18 and 79 in 2015.

Diabetes prevalence—which is the total number of existing cases, including new cases—among adults continues to go up (Figure 1.1). About 30.3 million people, or 9.4 percent of the U.S. population, had diabetes in 2015. This total included 30.2 million adults 18 years of age or older, or 12.2 percent of all U.S. adults. About 7.2 million of these adults had diabetes but were not aware that they had the disease or did not report that they had it. Although the prevalence of adults with diagnosed diabetes went up sharply during the 1990s, it appears to have been stabilizing since 2009 (Figure 1.1).

The increase in the number of adults with diabetes in the United States may be due in part to people with the disease living longer because of improvements in self-management practices and healthcare services. As of 2016, more than 4,100 diabetes self-management education and support (DSMES) programs were offered across the United States.

Diabetes self-management education and support (DSMES) programs are intended to improve preventive practices among people with diabetes. About 1.1 million people with diabetes participated in DSMES programs recognized by the American Diabetes Association (ADA) or accredited by the American Association of Diabetes Educators (AADE) in 2016.

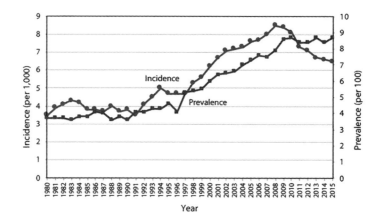

Figure 1.1. Trends in Incidence and Prevalence of Diagnosed Diabetes among Adults Aged 18 or Older, United States, 1980–2015

Race, Ethnicity, and Education

Members of some racial and ethnic minority groups are more likely to have diagnosed diabetes than non-Hispanic Whites. Among adults, American Indians/Alaska Natives had the highest age-adjusted rates of diagnosed diabetes among all racial and ethnic groups examined (Figure 1.2).

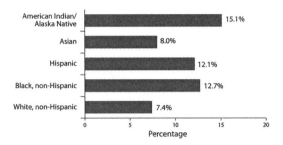

Figure 1.2. Percentage of U.S. Adults Aged 18 or Older with Diagnosed Diabetes, by Racial and Ethnic Group, 2013–2015 (Source: Figure adapted from the National Diabetes Statistics Report, 2017. Data sources: 2013–2015 National Health Interview Survey and 2015 Indian Health Service National Data Warehouse (American Indian/ Alaska Native data).)

Percentages are age-adjusted to the 2000 U.S. standard population.

A higher percentage of adults with less than a high-school education had diagnosed diabetes compared to adults with a high-school education or more than a high-school education (Figure 1.3).

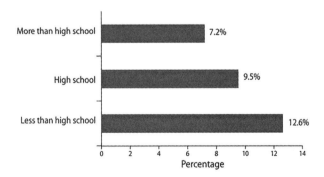

Figure 1.3. Percentage of U.S. Adults Aged 18 or Older with Diagnosed Diabetes, by Education Level, 2013–2015 (Source: Figure adapted from the National Diabetes Statistics Report, 2017. Data source: 2013–2015 National Health Interview Survey.)
Percentages are age-adjusted to the 2000 U.S. standard population.

A person's socioeconomic position is defined by her or his education and income level. Differences in diabetes prevalence were seen in the overall U.S. population and within racial and ethnic groups according to socioeconomic position. For example, the prevalence of diabetes increased among non-Hispanic Whites with less education and lower incomes and among Hispanics with less education. In addition, an association was found between lower education levels and less use of preventive care practices, such as annual foot and eye exams and regular monitoring of blood sugar levels.

Research suggests that the effectiveness of interventions designed to help people reduce their risk of type 2 diabetes and manage or prevent complications can vary by socioeconomic position. Healthy People 2020, the nation's agenda for improving the health of all Americans, and recent studies have identified socioeconomic position as an important factor to consider when evaluating the effectiveness of interventions.

Chapter 2

Who Is at Risk for Diabetes?

Prediabetes

You are at risk for developing prediabetes if you:

- Are overweight

- Are 45 years or older

- Have a parent, brother, or sister with type 2 diabetes

- Are physically active less than 3 times a week

- Have ever had gestational diabetes (diabetes during pregnancy) or given birth to a baby who weighed more than 9 pounds

- Are African American, Hispanic/Latino American, American Indian, or Alaska Native (some Pacific Islanders and Asian Americans are also at higher risk)

You can prevent or reverse prediabetes with simple, proven lifestyle changes such as losing weight if you are overweight, eating healthier, and getting regular physical activity.

Type 1 Diabetes

Type 1 diabetes is thought to be caused by an immune reaction (the body attacks itself by mistake). Risk factors for type 1 diabetes are not as clear as for prediabetes and type 2 diabetes. Known risk factors include:

About This Chapter: Text beginning with the heading "Type 1 Diabetes" is excerpted from "What are the Causes of Sinus Infections?" Centers for Disease Control and Prevention (CDC), July 25, 2017; Text under the heading "Family Health History and Diabetes" is excerpted from "Family Health History and Diabetes," Centers for Disease Control and Prevention (CDC), July 18, 2017.

- **Family history:** Having a parent, brother, or sister with type 1 diabetes
- **Age:** You can get type 1 diabetes at any age, but it is more likely to develop when you are a child, teen, or young adult.

In the United States, Whites are more likely to develop type 1 diabetes than African Americans and Hispanic/Latinx Americans.

Currently, no one knows how to prevent type 1 diabetes.

Type 2 Diabetes

You are at risk for developing type 2 diabetes if you:

- Have prediabetes
- Are overweight
- Are 45 years of age or older
- Have a parent, brother, or sister with type 2 diabetes
- Are physically active less than 3 times a week
- Have ever had gestational diabetes (diabetes during pregnancy) or given birth to a baby who weighed more than 9 pounds
- Are African American, Hispanic/Latinx American, American Indian, or Alaska Native (some Pacific Islanders and Asian Americans are also at a higher risk)

You can prevent or delay type 2 diabetes with simple, proven lifestyle changes, such as losing weight if you are overweight, eating healthier, and getting regular physical activity.

Gestational Diabetes

You are at risk for developing gestational diabetes (diabetes while pregnant) if you:

- Had gestational diabetes during a previous pregnancy
- Have given birth to a baby who weighed more than 9 pounds
- Are overweight
- Are more than 25 years of age
- Have a family history of type 2 diabetes

- Have a hormone disorder called "polycystic ovary syndrome" (PCOS)

- Are African American, Hispanic/Latinx American, American Indian, Alaska Native, Native Hawaiian, or Pacific Islander

Gestational diabetes usually goes away after your baby is born but increases your risk for type 2 diabetes later in life. Your baby is more likely to become obese as a child or teen, and they are more likely to develop type 2 diabetes later in life too.

Before you get pregnant, you may be able to prevent gestational diabetes by losing weight if you are overweight, eating healthier, and getting regular physical activity.

Family Health History and Diabetes

If you have a mother, father, sister, or brother with diabetes, you are more likely to get diabetes yourself. You are also more likely to have prediabetes. Talk to your doctor about your family health history of diabetes. Your doctor can help you take steps to prevent or delay diabetes, and reverse prediabetes if you have it.

Over 30 million people have diabetes. People with diabetes have levels of blood sugar that are too high. The different types of diabetes include type 1 diabetes, type 2 diabetes, and gestational diabetes. Diabetes can cause serious health problems, including heart disease, kidney problems, stroke, blindness, and the need for lower leg amputations.

Family History and Prediabetes

If you have a family health history of diabetes, you are more likely to have prediabetes and develop diabetes. You are also more likely to get type 2 diabetes if you have had gestational diabetes, are overweight or obese, or are African American, American Indian, Asian American, Pacific Islander, or Hispanic. Learning about your family health history of diabetes is an important step in finding out if you have prediabetes and knowing if you are more likely to get diabetes. Be sure to let your doctor know about your family health history of diabetes, especially if you have a mother, father, sister, or brother with diabetes. Your doctor might recommend that you have screening for diabetes earlier. Even if you have a family health history of diabetes, you can prevent or delay type 2 diabetes by eating healthier, being physically active, and maintaining or reaching a healthy weight. This is especially important if you have prediabetes, and taking these steps can reverse prediabetes.

People with prediabetes have levels of blood sugar that are higher than normal, but not high enough for them to be diagnosed with diabetes. People with prediabetes are more likely to get type 2 diabetes. About 84 million people in the United States have prediabetes, but most of them don't know they have it. If you have prediabetes, you can take steps to reverse it and prevent or delay diabetes—but not if you don't know that you have it.

Chapter 3

Diabetes in Children and Adolescents

Until now, the most common type of diabetes in children and teens has been type 1. It was called "juvenile diabetes." With type 1 diabetes, the pancreas does not make insulin. Insulin is a hormone that helps glucose, or sugar, get into your cells to give them energy. Without insulin, too much sugar stays in the blood.

Now, younger people are also getting type 2 diabetes. Type 2 diabetes used to be called "adult-onset diabetes." However, due to the rise of obesity, it is becoming more common in children and teens. With type 2 diabetes, the body does not make or use insulin well.

Children have a higher risk of type 2 diabetes if they are overweight or obese, have a family history of diabetes, or are not active. Children who are African American, Hispanic, Native American/Alaska Native, Asian American, or Pacific Islander also have a higher risk. To lower the risk of type 2 diabetes in children:

- Have them maintain a healthy weight
- Be sure they are physically active
- Have them eat smaller portions of healthy foods
- Limit their time with the TV, computer, and videos

About This Chapter: Text in this chapter begins with excerpts from "Diabetes in Children and Teens," MedlinePlus, National Institutes of Health (NIH), April 29, 2019; Text under the heading "Rates of New Diagnosed Cases of Type 1 and Type 2 Diabetes on the Rise among Children, Teens" is excerpted from "Rates of New Diagnosed Cases of Type 1 and Type 2 Diabetes on the Rise among Children, Teens," National Institutes of Health (NIH), April 13, 2017.

Children and teens with type 1 diabetes may need to take insulin. Type 2 diabetes may be controlled with diet and exercise. If not, patients will need to take oral diabetes medicines or insulin. A blood test called the "A1C" can check on how you are managing your diabetes.

Help Kids Stay Active to Prevent Diabetes

Children should participate in at least 60 minutes of moderate intensity physical activity most days of the week, preferably daily. Remember that children imitate adults. Start adding physical activity to your own daily routine and encourage your child to join you.

Some examples of moderate-intensity physical activity include:

- Brisk walking
- Playing tag
- Jumping rope
- Playing soccer
- Swimming
- Dancing

(Source: Excerpted from "Tips for Parents–Ideas to Help Children Maintain a Healthy Weight," Centers for Disease Control and Prevention (CDC).)

Rates of New Diagnosed Cases of Type 1 and Type 2 Diabetes on the Rise among Children, Teens

Rates of new diagnosed cases of type 1 and type 2 diabetes are increasing among youth in the United States, according to a report, "Incidence Trends of Type 1 and Type 2 Diabetes among Youths, 2002 to 2012," published in the *New England Journal of Medicine (NEJM)*.

In the United States, 29.1 million people are living with diagnosed or undiagnosed diabetes, and about 208,000 people younger than 20 years of age are living with diagnosed diabetes.

This study is the first ever to estimate trends in newly diagnosed cases of type 1 and type 2 diabetes in youth (those under the age of 20), from the 5 major racial/ethnic groups in the United States: non-Hispanic Whites, non-Hispanic Blacks, Hispanics, Asian Americans/Pacific Islanders, and Native Americans. However, the Native American youth who participated in the search study are not representative of all Native American youth in the United States. Thus, these rates cannot be generalized to all Native American youth nationwide.

The Diabetes in Youth study, funded by the Centers for Disease Control and Prevention (CDC) and the National Institutes of Health (NIH), found that from 2002 to 2012, incidence, or the rate, of newly diagnosed cases of type 1 diabetes in youth increased by about 1.8 percent each year. During the same period, the rate of newly diagnosed cases of type 2 diabetes increased even more quickly, at 4.8 percent. The study included 11,244 youth between the ages of 0 and 19 with type 1 diabetes and 2,846 youth between the ages of 10 and 19 with type 2.

"Because of the early age of onset and longer diabetes duration, youth are at risk for developing diabetes-related complications at a younger age. This profoundly lessens their quality of life, shortens their life expectancy, and increases healthcare costs," said Giuseppina Imperatore, M.D., Ph.D., an epidemiologist at the CDC's Division of Diabetes Translation (DDT), National Diabetes Center for Chronic Disease Prevention and Health Promotion.

The study results reflect the nation's first and only ongoing assessment of trends in type 1 and type 2 diabetes among youth and help identify how the epidemic is changing over time in Americans under the age of 20.

Key Diabetes Findings from the Report

- Across all racial/ethnic groups, the rate of newly diagnosed cases of type 1 diabetes increased more annually from 2003 to 2012 in males (2.2 percent) than in females (1.4 percent) between the ages of 0 and 19.

- Among youth between the ages of 0 and 19, the rate of newly diagnosed cases of type 1 diabetes increased most sharply in Hispanic youth, a 4.2 percent annual increase. In non-Hispanic Blacks, the rate of newly diagnosed cases of type 1 diabetes increased by 2.2 percent and in non-Hispanic Whites by 1.2 percent per year.

- Among youth between the ages of 10 and 19, the rate of newly diagnosed cases of type 2 diabetes rose most sharply in Native Americans (8.9 percent), Asian Americans/Pacific Islanders (8.5 percent), and non-Hispanic Blacks (6.3 percent).

Note: The rates for Native Americans cannot be generalized to all Native American youth nationwide.

- Among youth between the ages of 10 and 19, the rate of newly diagnosed cases of type 2 diabetes increased 3.1 percent among Hispanics. The smallest increase was seen in Whites (0.6 percent).

- The rate of newly diagnosed cases of type 2 diabetes rose much more sharply in females (6.2 percent) than in males (3.7 percent) between the ages of 10 and 19.

Cause of Rising Diabetes Incidence Unclear

"These findings lead to many more questions," said Barbara Linder, M.D., Ph.D., senior advisor for childhood diabetes research at the NIH's National Institute of Diabetes and Digestive and Kidney Diseases (NIDDK). "The differences among racial and ethnic groups and between genders raise many questions. We need to understand why the increase in rates of diabetes development varies so greatly and is so concentrated in specific racial and ethnic groups."

Type 1 diabetes, the most common form of diabetes in young people, is a condition in which the body fails to make insulin. Causes of type 1 diabetes are still unknown. However, disease development is suspected to follow exposure of genetically predisposed people to an "environmental trigger," stimulating an immune attack against the insulin-producing beta cells of the pancreas.

In type 2 diabetes, the body does not make or use insulin well. In the past, type 2 diabetes was extremely rare in youth, but it has become more common. Several NIH-funded studies are directly examining how to delay, prevent, and treat diabetes:

- Type 1 Diabetes TrialNet screens thousands of relatives of people with type 1 diabetes annually and conducts prevention studies with those at highest risk for the disease.

- The Environmental Determinants of Diabetes in the Young (TEDDY) study seeks to uncover factors that may increase the development of type 1 diabetes.

- For youth with type 2 diabetes, the ongoing Treatment Options for Type 2 Diabetes in Adolescents and Youth (TODAY) study is examining methods to treat the disease and prevent complications.

Chapter 4

Metabolic Syndrome: An Early Warning Sign

What Is Metabolic Syndrome?

"Metabolic syndrome" is the name for a group of risk factors that raises your risk for heart disease and other health problems, such as diabetes and stroke.

The term "metabolic" refers to the biochemical processes involved in the body's normal functioning. Risk factors are traits, conditions, or habits that increase your chance of developing a disease.

In this chapter, "heart disease" refers to ischemic heart disease, a condition in which a waxy substance called "plaque" builds up inside the arteries that supply blood to the heart.

Plaque hardens and narrows the arteries, reducing blood flow to your heart muscle. This can lead to chest pain, a heart attack, heart damage, or even death.

The five conditions described below are metabolic risk factors. You can have any one of these risk factors by itself, but they tend to occur together. You must have at least three metabolic risk factors to be diagnosed with metabolic syndrome.

- A large waistline. This also is called "abdominal obesity" or having an "apple shape." Excess fat in the stomach area is a greater risk factor for heart disease than excess fat in other parts of the body, such as on the hips.

- A high triglyceride level (or you are on medicine to treat high triglycerides). Triglycerides are a type of fat found in the blood.

About This Chapter: This chapter includes text excerpted from "Metabolic Syndrome," National Heart, Lung, and Blood Institute (NHLBI), January 30, 2019.

- A low high-density lipoprotein (HDL) cholesterol level (or you are on medicine to treat low HDL cholesterol). HDL sometimes is called "good" cholesterol. This is because it helps remove cholesterol from your arteries. A low HDL cholesterol level raises your risk for heart disease.

- High blood pressure (or you are on medicine to treat high blood pressure). Blood pressure is the force of blood pushing against the walls of your arteries as your heart pumps blood. If this pressure rises and stays high over time, it can damage your heart and lead to plaque buildup.

- High fasting blood sugar (or you are on medicine to treat high blood sugar). Mildly high blood sugar may be an early sign of diabetes.

Your risk for heart disease, diabetes, and stroke increases with the number of metabolic risk factors you have. The risk of having metabolic syndrome is closely linked to being overweight or obese and a lack of physical activity.

Insulin resistance also may increase your risk of metabolic syndrome. Insulin resistance is a condition in which the body cannot use its insulin properly. Insulin is a hormone that helps move blood sugar into cells where it is used for energy. Insulin resistance can lead to high blood sugar levels, and it is closely linked to being overweight or obese. Genetics (ethnicity and family history) and older age are other factors that may play a role in causing metabolic syndrome.

Metabolic syndrome is becoming more common due to a rise in obesity rates among adults. In the future, metabolic syndrome may overtake smoking as the leading risk factor for heart disease.

It is possible to prevent or delay metabolic syndrome, mainly with lifestyle changes. A healthy lifestyle is a lifelong commitment. Successfully controlling metabolic syndrome requires long-term effort and teamwork with your healthcare providers.

Other Names of Metabolic Syndrome

- Dysmetabolic syndrome
- Hypertriglyceridemic waist
- Insulin resistance syndrome
- Obesity syndrome
- Syndrome X

Causes of Metabolic Syndrome

Metabolic syndrome has several causes that act together. You can control some of the causes, such as being overweight or obese, an inactive lifestyle, and insulin resistance.

You cannot control other factors that may play a role in causing metabolic syndrome, such as growing older. Your risk for metabolic syndrome increases with age.

You also cannot control genetics (ethnicity and family history), which may play a role in causing the condition. For example, genetics can increase your risk of insulin resistance, which can lead to metabolic syndrome.

People who have metabolic syndrome often have two other conditions: Excessive blood clotting and constant, low-grade inflammation throughout the body. Researchers do not know whether these conditions cause metabolic syndrome or worsen it.

Researchers continue to study conditions that may play a role in metabolic syndrome, such as:

- A fatty liver (excess triglycerides and other fats in the liver)
- Polycystic ovarian syndrome (a tendency to develop cysts on the ovaries)
- Gallstones
- Breathing problems during sleep (such as sleep apnea)

Signs, Symptoms, and Complications of Metabolic Syndrome

Metabolic syndrome is a group of risk factors that raises your risk for heart disease and other health problems, such as diabetes and stroke. These risk factors can increase your risk for health problems even if they are only moderately raised (borderline-high risk factors).

Most of the metabolic risk factors have no signs or symptoms; although, a large waistline is a visible sign.

Some people may have symptoms of high blood sugar if diabetes—especially type 2 diabetes—is present. Symptoms of high blood sugar often include increased thirst; increased urination, especially at night; fatigue (tiredness); and blurred vision.

High blood pressure usually has no signs or symptoms. However, some people in the early stages of high blood pressure may have dull headaches, dizzy spells, or more nosebleeds than usual.

Risk Factors of Metabolic Syndrome

People at the greatest risk for metabolic syndrome have these underlying causes:

- Abdominal obesity (a large waistline)

- An inactive lifestyle

- Insulin resistance

Some people are at risk for metabolic syndrome because they take medicines that cause weight gain or changes in blood pressure, blood cholesterol, and blood sugar levels. These medicines most often are used to treat inflammation, allergies, human immunodeficiency virus (HIV), and depression and other types of mental illness.

Populations Affected

Some racial and ethnic groups in the United States are at a higher risk for metabolic syndrome than others. Mexican Americans have the highest rate of metabolic syndrome, followed by Whites and Blacks.

Other groups at an increased risk for metabolic syndrome include:

- People who have a personal history of diabetes

- People who have a sibling or parent who has diabetes

- Women

- Women who have a personal history of polycystic ovarian syndrome

Heart Disease Risk

Metabolic syndrome increases your risk for ischemic heart disease. Other risk factors, besides metabolic syndrome, also increase your risk for heart disease. For example, a high low-density lipoprotein (LDL) ("bad") cholesterol level and smoking are major risk factors for heart disease.

Even if you do not have metabolic syndrome, you should find out your short-term risk for heart disease. The National Cholesterol Education Program (NCEP) divides short-term heart disease risk into four categories. Your risk category depends on which risk factors you have and how many you have.

Your risk factors are used to calculate your 10-year risk of developing heart disease. The NCEP has an online calculator that you can use to estimate your 10-year risk of having a heart attack.

- **High risk**: You are in this category if you already have heart disease or diabetes, or if your 10-year risk score is more than 20 percent.

- **Moderately high risk**: You are in this category if you have 2 or more risk factors and your 10-year risk score is 10 percent to 20 percent.

- **Moderate risk**: You are in this category if you have 2 or more risk factors and your 10-year risk score is less than 10 percent.

- **Lower risk**: You are in this category if you have zero or one risk factor.

Even if your 10-year risk score is not high, metabolic syndrome will increase your risk for coronary heart disease over time.

Screening and Prevention of Metabolic Syndrome

The best way to prevent metabolic syndrome is to adopt heart-healthy lifestyle changes. Make sure to schedule routine doctor visits to keep track of your cholesterol, blood pressure, and blood sugar levels. Speak with your doctor about a blood test called a "lipoprotein panel," which shows your levels of total cholesterol, LDL cholesterol, HDL cholesterol, and triglycerides.

Diagnosis of Metabolic Syndrome

Your doctor will diagnose metabolic syndrome based on the results of a physical exam and blood tests. You must have at least three of the five metabolic risk factors to be diagnosed with metabolic syndrome.

Metabolic Risk Factors
A Large Waistline

Having a large waistline means that you carry excess weight around your waist. This is also called having an "apple-shaped" figure. Your doctor will measure your waist to find out whether you have a large waistline.

A waist measurement of 35 inches or more for women or 40 inches or more for men is a metabolic risk factor. A large waistline means that you are at an increased risk for heart disease and other health problems.

A High Triglyceride Level

Triglycerides are a type of fat found in the blood. A triglyceride level of 150 mg/dL or higher (or being on medicine to treat high triglycerides) is a metabolic risk factor. (The mg/dL is milligrams per deciliter—the units used to measure triglycerides, cholesterol, and blood sugar.)

A Low High-Density Lipoprotein Cholesterol Level

High-density lipoprotein cholesterol sometimes is called "good" cholesterol. This is because it helps remove cholesterol from your arteries.

A high-density lipoprotein cholesterol level of less than 50 mg/dL for women and less than 40 mg/dL for men (or being on medicine to treat low HDL cholesterol) is a metabolic risk factor.

High Blood Pressure

A blood pressure of 130/85 mmHg or higher (or being on medicine to treat high blood pressure) is a metabolic risk factor. (The mmHg is millimeters of mercury—the units used to measure blood pressure.)

If only one of your two blood pressure numbers is high, you are still at risk for metabolic syndrome.

High Fasting Blood Sugar

A normal fasting blood sugar level is less than 100 mg/dL. A fasting blood sugar level between 100–125 mg/dL is considered prediabetes. A fasting blood sugar level of 126 mg/dL or higher is considered diabetes.

A fasting blood sugar level of 100 mg/dL or higher (or being on medicine to treat high blood sugar) is a metabolic risk factor.

About 85 percent of people who have type 2 diabetes—the most common type of diabetes—also have metabolic syndrome. These people have a much higher risk for heart disease than the 15 percent of people who have type 2 diabetes without metabolic syndrome.

Treatment of Metabolic Syndrome

Heart-healthy lifestyle changes are the first line of treatment for metabolic syndrome. If heart-healthy lifestyle changes are not enough, your doctor may prescribe medicines. Medicines are used to treat and control risk factors, such as high blood pressure, high triglycerides, low HDL cholesterol, and high blood sugar.

Goals of Treatment

The major goal of treating metabolic syndrome is to reduce the risk of ischemic heart disease. Treatment is directed first at lowering LDL cholesterol and high blood pressure and managing diabetes (if these conditions are present).

The second goal of treatment is to prevent the onset of type 2 diabetes, if it has not already developed. Long-term complications of diabetes often include heart and kidney disease, vision loss, and foot or leg amputation. If diabetes is present, the goal of treatment is to reduce your risk of heart disease by controlling all of your risk factors.

Heart-Healthy Lifestyle Changes

Heart-healthy lifestyle changes include heart-healthy eating, aiming for a healthy weight, managing stress, physical activity, and quitting smoking.

Medicines

Sometimes, lifestyle changes are not enough to control your risk factors for metabolic syndrome. For example, you may need statin medications to control or lower your cholesterol. By lowering your blood cholesterol level, you can decrease your chance of having a heart attack or stroke. Doctors usually prescribe statins for people who have:

- Diabetes

- Heart disease or had a prior stroke

- High LDL cholesterol levels

Doctors may discuss beginning statin treatment with those who have an elevated risk for developing heart disease or having a stroke.

Your doctor also may prescribe other medications to:

- Decrease your chance of having a heart attack or dying suddenly

- Lower your blood pressure

- Prevent blood clots, which can lead to heart attack or stroke

- Reduce your heart's workload, and relieve symptoms of coronary heart disease

Take all medicines regularly, as your doctor prescribes. Do not change the amount of your medicine or skip a dose unless your doctor tells you to. You should still follow a heart-healthy lifestyle, even if you take medicines to treat your risk factors for metabolic syndrome.

The Role of Diet in Metabolic Syndrome

Dr. Lyn M. Steffen at the University of Minnesota's School of Public Health and her colleagues set out to take a broad look at the relationship between metabolic syndrome and dietary intake. They used data from 9,514 middle-aged adults enrolled in the multicenter Atherosclerosis Risk in Communities (ARIC) study. The study was initiated by NIH's National Heart, Lung and Blood Institute (NHLBI) to investigate the factors that contribute to atherosclerosis (the buildup of cholesterol and fat in the walls of arteries) and the incidence of cardiovascular diseases.

The study found that a Western dietary pattern characterized by high intakes of refined grains, processed meat, fried foods, and red meat—was associated with a greater risk of developing metabolic syndrome. Upon closer analysis, the researchers found that those who ate the most meat were more likely to develop metabolic syndrome. In particular, hamburgers, hot dogs, and processed meats were each associated with higher rates of metabolic syndrome. Fried foods were also associated with an increased risk.

The researchers did not find any association, positive or negative, between metabolic syndrome and whole grains, refined grains, nuts, coffee or fruits and vegetables. On the other hand, they found that those who ate more dairy were less likely to develop metabolic syndrome.

(Source: "The Role of Diet in Metabolic Syndrome," National Institutes of Health (NIH).)

Living with Metabolic Syndrome

Metabolic syndrome is a lifelong condition. However, lifestyle changes can help you control your risk factors and reduce your risk for ischemic heart disease and diabetes.

If you already have heart disease or diabetes, lifestyle changes can help you prevent or delay related problems. Examples of these problems include heart attack, stroke, and diabetes-related complications (for example, damage to your eyes, nerves, kidneys, feet, and legs).

Heart-healthy lifestyle changes may include:

- Heart-healthy eating

- Aiming for a healthy weight

- Managing stress

- Physical activity

- Quitting smoking

If lifestyle changes are not enough, your doctor may recommend medicines. Take all of your medicines as prescribed by your doctor. Make realistic short- and long-term goals for yourself when you begin to make healthy lifestyle changes. Work closely with your doctor, and seek regular medical care.

Chapter 5

Insulin Resistance and Prediabetes

What Is Insulin?

Insulin is a hormone made by the pancreas that helps glucose in your blood enter cells in your muscle, fat, and liver, where it is used for energy. Glucose comes from the food you eat. The liver also makes glucose in times of need, such as when you are fasting. When blood glucose, also called "blood sugar," levels rise after you eat, your pancreas releases insulin into the blood. Insulin then lowers blood glucose to keep it in the normal range.

What Is Insulin Resistance?

Insulin resistance is when cells in your muscles, fat, and liver do not respond well to insulin and cannot easily take up glucose from your blood. As a result, your pancreas makes more insulin to help glucose enter your cells. As long as your pancreas can make enough insulin to overcome your cells' weak response to insulin, your blood glucose levels will stay in the healthy range.

What Is Prediabetes?

Prediabetes means that your blood glucose levels are higher than normal but not high enough to be diagnosed as diabetes. Prediabetes usually occurs in people who already have some insulin resistance or whose beta cells in the pancreas are not making enough insulin to

About This Chapter: This chapter includes text excerpted from "Insulin Resistance and Prediabetes," National Institute of Diabetes and Digestive and Kidney Diseases (NIDDK), May 2018.

keep blood glucose in the normal range. Without enough insulin, extra glucose stays in your bloodstream rather than entering your cells. Over time, you could develop type 2 diabetes.

Insulin in a Nutshell

This vital hormone—you can't survive without it—regulates blood sugar (glucose) in the body, a very complicated process. Here are the high points:

- The food you eat is broken down into glucose.
- Glucose enters your bloodstream, which signals the pancreas to release insulin.
- Insulin helps glucose enter the body's cells so it can be used for energy.
- Insulin also signals the liver to store glucose for later use.
- Glucose enters cells, and glucose levels in the bloodstream decrease, signaling insulin to decrease too.
- Lower insulin levels alert the liver to release stored glucose so energy is always available, even if you haven't eaten for a while.

That's when everything works smoothly. But this finely tuned system can quickly get out of whack, as follows:

- A lot of glucose enters the bloodstream.
- The pancreas pumps out more insulin to get glucose into cells.
- Over time, cells stop responding to all that insulin—they've become insulin resistant.
- The pancreas keeps making more insulin to try to make cells respond.
- Eventually, the pancreas can't keep up, and glucose keeps rising.

(Source: "Diabetes: What's Insulin Resistance Got to Do with It?" Centers for Disease Control and Prevention (CDC).)

Who Is More Likely to Develop Insulin Resistance or Prediabetes?

People who have genetic or lifestyle risk factors are more likely to develop insulin resistance or prediabetes. Risk factors include:

- Being overweight or obese
- Being 45 years of age or older
- Having a parent, brother, or sister with diabetes

- Being of African American, Alaska Native, American Indian, Asian American, Hispanic/Latinx, Native Hawaiian, or Pacific Islander American ethnicity

- Being physically inactive

- Having other health conditions, such as high blood pressure and abnormal cholesterol levels

- Having a history of gestational diabetes

- Having a history of heart disease or stroke

- Having polycystic ovary syndrome (PCOS)

People who have metabolic syndrome—a combination of high blood pressure, abnormal cholesterol levels, and large waist size—are more likely to have prediabetes.

Along with these risk factors, other things that may contribute to insulin resistance include:

- Certain medicines, such as glucocorticoids, some antipsychotics, and some medicines for human immunodeficiency viruses (HIV)

- Hormonal disorders, such as Cushing syndrome and acromegaly

- Sleep problems, especially sleep apnea

Although you cannot change risk factors such as family history, age, or ethnicity, you can change lifestyle risk factors around eating, physical activity, and weight. These lifestyle changes can lower your chances of developing insulin resistance or prediabetes.

How Common Is Prediabetes

More than 84 million people 18 years of age and older have prediabetes in the United States. That is about 1 out of every 3 adults.

What Causes Insulin Resistance and Prediabetes

Researchers do not fully understand what causes insulin resistance and prediabetes, but they think that excess weight and a lack of physical activity are major factors.

Excess Weight

Experts believe that obesity, especially too much fat in the abdomen and around the organs, called "visceral fat," is the main cause of insulin resistance. A waist measurement of 40 inches or more for men and 35 inches or more for women is linked to insulin resistance. This is true even if your body mass index (BMI) falls within the normal range. However, research has shown that Asian Americans may have an increased risk for insulin resistance even without a high BMI.

Researchers used to think that fat tissue was only for energy storage. However, studies have shown that belly fat makes hormones and other substances that can contribute to chronic, or long-lasting, inflammation in the body. Inflammation may play a role in insulin resistance, type 2 diabetes, and cardiovascular disease (CVD).

Excess weight may lead to insulin resistance, which may play a part in the development of the fatty liver disease.

Physical Inactivity

Not getting enough physical activity is linked to insulin resistance and prediabetes. Regular physical activity causes changes in your body that make it better able to keep your blood glucose levels in balance.

What Are the Symptoms of Insulin Resistance and Prediabetes?

Insulin resistance and prediabetes usually have no symptoms. Some people with prediabetes may have darkened skin in the armpits or on the back and sides of the neck, a condition called "acanthosis nigricans." Many small skin growths called "skin tags" often appear in these same areas.

Even though blood glucose levels are not high enough to cause symptoms for most people, a few research studies have shown that some people with prediabetes may already have early changes in their eyes that can lead to retinopathy. This problem more often occurs in people with diabetes.

How Do Doctors Diagnose Insulin Resistance and Prediabetes?

Doctors use blood tests to find out if someone has prediabetes, but they do not usually test for insulin resistance. The most accurate test for insulin resistance is complicated and used mostly for research.

Doctors most often use the fasting plasma glucose (FPG) test or the A1C test to diagnose prediabetes. Less often, doctors use the oral glucose tolerance test (OGTT), which is more expensive and not as easy to give.

The A1C test reflects your average blood glucose over the past three months. The FPG and OGTT show your blood glucose level at the time of the test. The A1C test is not as sensitive as the other tests. In some people, it may miss prediabetes that the OGTT could catch. The OGTT can identify how your body handles glucose after a meal—often before your fasting blood glucose level becomes abnormal. Often, doctors use the OGTT to check for gestational diabetes, a type of diabetes that develops during pregnancy.

People with prediabetes have up to a 50 percent chance of developing diabetes over the next 5 to 10 years. You can take steps to manage your prediabetes and prevent type 2 diabetes.

The following test results show prediabetes:

- A1C—5.7 to 6.4 percent

- FPG—100 to 125 mg/dL (milligrams per deciliter)

- OGTT—140 to 199 mg/dL

You should be tested for prediabetes if you are overweight or obese and have one or more other risk factors for diabetes, or if your parents, siblings, or children have type 2 diabetes. Even if you do not have risk factors, you should start getting tested once you reach the age of 45.

If the results are normal but you have other risk factors for diabetes, you should be retested at least every three years.

How Can I Prevent or Reverse Insulin Resistance and Prediabetes?

Physical activity and losing weight if you need to may help your body respond better to insulin. Taking small steps, such as eating healthier foods and moving more to lose weight, can help reverse insulin resistance and prevent or delay type 2 diabetes in people with prediabetes.

The Diabetes Prevention Program (DPP), a study funded by the National Institutes of Health (NIH), showed that for people at high risk of developing diabetes, losing 5 to 7 percent of their starting weight helped reduce their chance of developing the disease. That is 10 to 14 pounds for someone who weighs 200 pounds. People in the study lost weight by changing their diet and being more physically active.

The Diabetes Prevention Program also showed that taking metformin, a medicine used to treat diabetes, could delay diabetes. Metformin worked best for women with a history of gestational diabetes, younger adults, and people with obesity. Ask your doctor if metformin might be right for you.

Making a plan, tracking your progress, and getting support from your healthcare professional, family, and friends can help you make lifestyle changes that may prevent or reverse insulin resistance and prediabetes. You may be able to take part in a lifestyle change program as part of the National Diabetes Prevention Program (NDPP).

Chapter 6

Type 1 Diabetes

What Is Type 1 Diabetes?

Diabetes occurs when your blood glucose, also called "blood sugar," is too high. Blood glucose is your main source of energy and comes mainly from the food you eat. Insulin, a hormone made by the pancreas, helps the glucose in your blood get into your cells to be used for energy. Another hormone, glucagon, works with insulin to control blood glucose levels.

In most people with type 1 diabetes, the body's immune system, which normally fights infection, attacks and destroys the cells in the pancreas that make insulin. As a result, your pancreas stops making insulin. Without insulin, glucose cannot get into your cells, and your blood glucose rises above normal. People with type 1 diabetes need to take insulin every day to stay alive.

Who Is More Likely to Develop Type 1 Diabetes?

Type 1 diabetes typically occurs in children and young adults, although it can appear at any age. Having a parent or sibling with the disease may increase your chance of developing type 1 diabetes. In the United States, about five percent of people with diabetes have type 1.

About This Chapter: This chapter includes text excerpted from "Type 1 Diabetes," National Institute of Diabetes and Digestive and Kidney Diseases (NIDDK), July 2017.

> **Other Names for Type 1 Diabetes**
> - Autoimmune diabetes
> - Diabetes mellitus type 1
> - Insulin-dependent diabetes mellitus (IDDM)
> - Juvenile diabetes
> - Juvenile-onset diabetes (JOD)
> - Juvenile-onset diabetes mellitus
> - T1D
> - Type 1 diabetes mellitus
>
> *(Source: "Type 1 Diabetes," Genetics Home Reference (GHR), National Institutes of Health (NIH).)*

What Are the Symptoms of Type 1 Diabetes?

Symptoms of type 1 diabetes are serious and usually happen quickly, over a few days to a few weeks. Symptoms can include:

- Increased thirst and urination
- Increased hunger
- Blurred vision
- Fatigue
- Unexplained weight loss

Sometimes, the first symptoms of type 1 diabetes are signs of a life-threatening condition called "diabetic ketoacidosis" (DKA). Some symptoms of DKA include:

- Breath that smells fruity
- Dry or flushed skin
- Nausea or vomiting
- Stomach pain
- Trouble breathing
- Trouble paying attention or feeling confused

Diabetic ketoacidosis is serious and dangerous. If you or your child have symptoms of DKA, contact your healthcare professional right away, or go to the nearest hospital emergency room.

What Causes Type 1 Diabetes

Experts think that type 1 diabetes is caused by genes and factors in the environment, such as viruses, that might trigger the disease. Researchers are working to pinpoint the causes of type 1 diabetes through studies, such as TrialNet.

Frequency of Type 1 Diabetes

Type 1 diabetes occurs in 10 to 20 per 100,000 people per year in the United States. By age 18, approximately 1 in 300 people in the United States develop type 1 diabetes. The disorder occurs with similar frequencies in Europe, the United Kingdom, Canada, and New Zealand. Type 1 diabetes occurs much less frequently in Asia and South America, with reported incidences as low as 1 in 1 million per year. For unknown reasons, during the past 20 years the worldwide incidence of type 1 diabetes has been increasing by 2 to 5 percent each year.

Type 1 diabetes accounts for 5 to 10 percent of cases of diabetes worldwide. Most people with diabetes have type 2 diabetes, in which the body continues to produce insulin but becomes less able to use it.

(Source: "Type 1 Diabetes," Genetics Home Reference (GHR), National Institutes of Health (NIH).)

How Do Healthcare Professionals Diagnose Type 1 Diabetes?

Healthcare professionals usually test people for type 1 diabetes if they have clear-cut diabetes symptoms. Healthcare professionals most often use the random plasma glucose (RPG) test to diagnose type 1 diabetes. This blood test measures your blood glucose level at a single point in time. Sometimes, health professionals also use the A1C blood test to find out how long someone has had high blood glucose.

Even though these tests can confirm that you have diabetes, they cannot identify what type you have. Treatment depends on the type of diabetes, so knowing whether you have type 1 or type 2 is important.

To find out if your diabetes is type 1, your healthcare professional may test your blood for certain autoantibodies. Autoantibodies are antibodies that attack your healthy tissues and cells by mistake. The presence of certain types of autoantibodies is common in type 1 but not in type 2 diabetes.

Because type 1 diabetes can run in families, your healthcare professional can test your family members for autoantibodies. TrialNet, an international research network, also offers autoantibody testing to family members of people diagnosed with the disease. The presence of autoantibodies, even without diabetes symptoms, means that the family member is more likely to develop type 1 diabetes. If you have a brother or sister, child, or parent with type 1 diabetes, you may want to get an autoantibody test. People 20 years of age or younger who have a cousin, aunt, uncle, niece, nephew, grandparent, or half-sibling with type 1 diabetes also may want to get tested.

What Medicines Do I Need to Treat My Type 1 Diabetes?

If you have type 1 diabetes, you must take insulin because your body no longer makes this hormone. Different types of insulin start to work at different speeds, and the effects of each last a different length of time. You may need to use more than one type. You can take insulin a number of ways. Common options include a needle and syringe, insulin pen, or insulin pump.

Some people who have trouble reaching their blood glucose targets with insulin alone also might need to take another type of diabetes medicine that works with insulin, such as pramlintide. Pramlintide, given by injection, helps keep blood glucose levels from going too high after eating. Few people with type 1 diabetes take pramlintide, however. The National Institutes of Health (NIH) has funded a large research study to test the use of pramlintide along with insulin and glucagon in people with type 1 diabetes. Another diabetes medicine, metformin, may help decrease the amount of insulin you need to take, but more studies are needed to confirm this. Researchers are also studying other diabetes pills that people with type 1 diabetes might take along with insulin.

Hypoglycemia, or low blood sugar, can occur if you take insulin but do not match your dose with your food or physical activity. Severe hypoglycemia can be dangerous and needs to be treated right away.

How Else Can I Manage Type 1 Diabetes?

Along with insulin and any other medicines you use, you can manage your diabetes by taking care of yourself each day. Following your diabetes meal plan, being physically active, and checking your blood glucose often are some of the ways you can take care of yourself. Work with your healthcare team to come up with a diabetes care plan that works for you. If you are planning a pregnancy and have been diagnosed with diabetes, try to get your blood glucose levels in your target range before you get pregnant.

Do I Have Other Treatment Options for My Type 1 Diabetes?

The National Institute of Diabetes and Digestive and Kidney Diseases (NIDDK) has played an important role in developing artificial pancreas technology. An artificial pancreas replaces manual blood glucose testing and the use of insulin shots. A single system monitors blood glucose levels around the clock and provides insulin or a combination of insulin and glucagon automatically. The system can also be monitored remotely, for example by parents or medical staff.

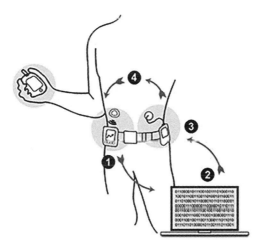

1. Continuous Glucose Monitor
2. Computer-Controlled Algorithm
3. Insulin Pump
4. Patient Effect

Figure 6.1. Artificial Pancreas Device System

An artificial pancreas system uses a continuous glucose monitor, an insulin pump, and a control algorithm to give you the right amount of basal insulin.

In 2016, the U.S. Food and Drug Administration (FDA) approved a type of artificial pancreas system called a "hybrid closed-loop system." This system tests your glucose level every five minutes throughout the day and night through a continuous glucose monitor, and it automatically gives you the right amount of basal insulin, a long-acting insulin, through a separate insulin pump. You still need to manually adjust the amount of insulin the pump delivers at mealtimes and when you need a correction dose. You also will need to test your blood with a glucose meter several times a day.

The continuous glucose monitor sends information through a software program called a "control algorithm." Based on your glucose level, the algorithm tells the insulin pump how much insulin to deliver. The software program could be installed on the pump or another device, such as a cell phone or computer.

Starting in late 2016 and early 2017, the NIDDK funded several important studies on different types of artificial pancreas devices to better help people with type 1 diabetes manage their disease. The devices may also help people with type 2 diabetes and gestational diabetes.

The NIDDK is also supporting research into pancreatic islet transplantation—an experimental treatment for hard-to-control type 1 diabetes. Pancreatic islets are clusters of cells in the pancreas that make insulin. Type 1 diabetes attacks these cells. A pancreatic islet transplant replaces destroyed islets with new ones that make and release insulin. This procedure takes islets from the pancreas of an organ donor and transfers them to a person with type 1 diabetes.

What Health Problems Can People with Type 1 Diabetes Develop?

Over time, high blood glucose leads to problems such as:

- Heart disease

- Stroke

- Kidney disease

- Eye problems

- Dental disease

- Nerve damage

- Foot problems

- Depression

- Sleep apnea

If you have type 1 diabetes, you can help prevent or delay the health problems of diabetes by managing your blood glucose, blood pressure, and cholesterol, and by following your self-care plan.

Can I Lower My Chance of Developing Type 1 Diabetes?

At this time, type 1 diabetes cannot be prevented. However, through studies such as TrialNet, researchers are working to identify possible ways to prevent or slow down the disease.

Chapter 7

Type 2 Diabetes

What Is Type 2 Diabetes?

Type 2 diabetes, the most common type of diabetes, is a disease that occurs when your blood glucose, also called "blood sugar," is too high. Blood glucose is your main source of energy and comes mainly from the food you eat. Insulin, a hormone made by the pancreas, helps glucose get into your cells to be used for energy. In type 2 diabetes, your body does not make enough insulin or does not use insulin well. Too much glucose then stays in your blood, and not enough reaches your cells.

The good news is that you can take steps to prevent or delay the development of type 2 diabetes.

Who Is More Likely to Develop Type 2 Diabetes?

You can develop type 2 diabetes at any age, even during childhood. However, type 2 diabetes occurs most often in middle-aged and older people. You are more likely to develop type 2 diabetes if you are 45 years of age or older, have a family history of diabetes, or are overweight or obese. Diabetes is more common in people who are African American, Hispanic/Latinx, American Indian, Asian American, or Pacific Islander.

Physical inactivity and certain health problems, such as high blood pressure, affect your chances of developing type 2 diabetes. You are also more likely to develop type 2 diabetes if you have prediabetes or had gestational diabetes when you were pregnant.

About This Chapter: This chapter includes text excerpted from "Type 2 Diabetes," National Institute of Diabetes and Digestive and Kidney Diseases (NIDDK), May 2017.

What Are the Symptoms of Diabetes?

Symptoms of diabetes include:

- Increased thirst and urination

- Increased hunger

- Feeling tired

- Blurred vision

- Numbness or tingling in the feet or hands

- Sores that do not heal

- Unexplained weight loss

Symptoms of type 2 diabetes often develop slowly—over the course of several years—and can be so mild that you might not even notice them. Many people have no symptoms. Some people do not find out they have the disease until they have diabetes-related health problems, such as blurred vision or heart disease.

What Causes Type 2 Diabetes

Type 2 diabetes is caused by several factors, including:

- Being overweight or obese

- Not being physically active

- Insulin resistance

- Genes

How Do Healthcare Professionals Diagnose Type 2 Diabetes?

Your healthcare professional can diagnose type 2 diabetes based on blood tests.

How Can I Manage My Type 2 Diabetes?

Managing your blood glucose, blood pressure, and cholesterol, and quitting smoking if you smoke, are important ways to manage your type 2 diabetes. Lifestyle changes that include planning healthy meals, limiting calories if you are overweight, and being physically active are also part of managing your diabetes. So is taking any prescribed medicines. Work with your healthcare team to create a diabetes care plan that works for you.

Genes and Family History

Certain genes may make you more likely to develop type 2 diabetes. The disease tends to run in families and occurs more often in these racial/ethnic groups:

- African Americans
- Alaska Natives
- American Indians
- Asian Americans
- Hispanics/Latins
- Native Hawaiians
- Pacific Islanders

Genes also can increase the risk of type 2 diabetes by increasing a person's tendency to become overweight or obese.

(Source: "Symptoms and Causes of Diabetes," National Institute of Diabetes and Digestive and Kidney Diseases (NIDDK).)

What Medicines Do I Need to Treat My Type 2 Diabetes?

Along with following your diabetes care plan, you may need diabetes medicines, which may include pills or medicines you inject under your skin, such as insulin. Over time, you may need more than one diabetes medicine to manage your blood glucose. Even if you do not take insulin, you may need it at special times, such as during pregnancy or if you are in the hospital. You also may need medicines for high blood pressure, high cholesterol, or other conditions.

What Health Problems Can People with Diabetes Develop?

Following a good diabetes care plan can help protect against many diabetes-related health problems. However, if it is not managed, diabetes can lead to problems such as:

- Heart disease and stroke

- Nerve damage

- Kidney disease

- Foot problems

- Eye disease

- Gum disease and other dental problems

- Sexual and bladder problems

Many people with type 2 diabetes also have nonalcoholic fatty liver disease (NAFLD). Losing weight if you are overweight or obese can improve NAFLD. Diabetes is also linked to other health problems, such as sleep apnea, depression, some types of cancer, and dementia.

You can take steps to lower your chances of developing these diabetes-related health problems.

How Can I Lower My Chances of Developing Type 2 Diabetes?

Research, such as the Diabetes Prevention Program (DPP), sponsored by the National Institutes of Health (NIH), has shown that you can take steps to reduce your chances of developing type 2 diabetes if you have risk factors for the disease. Here are some things you can do to lower your risk:

- **Lose weight if you are overweight, and keep it off.** You may be able to prevent or delay diabetes by losing 5 to 7 percent of your current weight. For instance, if you weigh 200 pounds, your goal would be to lose about 10 to 14 pounds.

- **Move more.** Get at least 30 minutes of physical activity, such as walking, at least 5 days a week. If you have not been active, talk with your healthcare professional about which activities are best. Start slowly and build up to your goal.

- **Eat healthy foods.** Eat smaller portions to reduce the amount of calories you eat each day to help you lose weight. Choosing foods with less fat is another way to reduce calories. Drink water instead of sweetened beverages.

Ask your healthcare team what other changes you can make to prevent or delay type 2 diabetes.

Most often, your best chance for preventing type 2 diabetes is to make lifestyle changes that work for you in the long term.

Chapter 8

Double Diabetes

What Is Double Diabetes?

Double diabetes, or "hybrid diabetes," is a condition that occurs when you have both type 1 and type 2 diabetes. Even though the harmful effects of type 1 diabetes persist, the effects of type 2 diabetes can be reduced over time. About 20.8 million Americans are believed to be diabetic. Among them, 6.2 million people have this disease. About 41 million people are prediabetic, a condition in which blood-glucose levels are higher than normal.

Causes of Double Diabetes

Type 1 diabetes is caused by your body producing little or no insulin, which is a hormone that regulates the amount of blood sugar, also known as "glucose," in your system. Type 2 diabetes forms if your body does not make enough insulin or if your body does not use insulin well because of the development of insulin resistance. The most common cause of type 2 diabetes is obesity. If you have type 1 diabetes and your family members have type 2 diabetes or vice versa, it is likely that you may be at risk of developing both types of diabetes.

Symptoms of Double Diabetes

The symptoms of double diabetes are the same as those of type 1 and type 2 diabetes.

About This Chapter: "Double Diabetes," © 2019 Omnigraphics. Reviewed June 2019.

Type 1 Diabetes

The symptoms of type 1 diabetes do not appear until the insulin-producing beta cells are destroyed to a point in which insulin production bottoms out. The most common symptoms of type 1 diabetes include:

- Frequent urination
- Extreme hunger
- Unusual thirst (especially for cold and sweet drinks)
- Weight loss (sudden or dramatic)
- Extreme fatigue
- Nausea and vomiting
- Blurred vision or changes in the eyesight

Type 2 Diabetes

The most common symptoms of type 2 diabetes are as follows:

- Fatigue
- Gum problems
- Itching
- Unusual sensations, such as tingling or burning
- Erectile dysfunction (ED) in men
- Vaginal yeast infections
- Fungal infections under the breast or groin in women

Diagnosis of Double Diabetes

The diagnostic procedures for both type 1 and type 2 diabetes are the same. The presence of diabetes can be diagnosed using the following tests:

- **Fasting plasma glucose (FPG) test:** The FPG test is the standard test for diagnosing diabetes and is conducted after eight hours of fasting. The FPG test is not reliable after only one test, so two or more tests are done if the first one points to diabetes.

- **Hemoglobin A1C test:** This test is used for examining the blood levels of glycosylated hemoglobin, also known as "hemoglobin A1C." The test results indicate the glucose level of your blood over the last two to three months. Specifically, this test measures the amount of blood sugar present in hemoglobin, an oxygen-carrying protein in the red blood cells.

- **Autoantibody test:** This test is conducted in order to detect any antibody-killing cells, known as "autoantibodies." The autoantibody test results can help differentiate between type 1 and type 2 diabetes.

- **Oral glucose tolerance test (OGTT):** The OGTT is only recommended after the FPG test as it may overdiagnose diabetes even if you do not have diabetes.

- An **electrocardiogram (ECG or EKG)** and other tests are recommended to check the presence of any heart-related diseases.

Treatment of Double Diabetes
Type 1 Diabetes

Treatment for type 1 diabetes is lifelong and requires frequent blood sugar monitoring and insulin therapy. The main goal of type 1 diabetes treatment is to keep your glucose levels as normal as possible in order to delay or prevent further complications. Ideally, your blood sugar levels should be between 80 and 130 mg/dL before meals, and your after-meal blood sugar level should not be more than 180 mg/dL. The types of insulin therapy include:

- Short-acting insulin
- Rapid-acting insulin
- Intermediate-acting insulin
- Long-acting insulin

Insulin cannot be taken orally because your stomach enzymes will break down the insulin entering your body, which further prevents its action. You can take insulin through injections or through insulin pumps. Depending upon the type of insulin therapy you take, it is recommended to check your blood glucose levels at least four times a day. Continuous glucose monitoring (CGM) can be used to monitor glucose levels throughout the day, and this can help prevent hypoglycemia.

Type 2 Diabetes

Treatment for type 2 diabetes includes the following:

Healthy eating: There is no specific diet plan for minimizing type 2 diabetes; however, you can better your diet by:

- Reducing calories

- Eating fewer sweets and refined food products

- Consuming more vegetables and fruits

- Eating more fiber-filled foods

Physical activity: It is recommended to consult your doctor before starting any exercises for treating type 2 diabetes. You can participate in physical activities, such as swimming, biking, and walking, for at least 30 to 60 minutes a day, which can help you lower your blood sugar levels and maintain them.

Losing weight: Losing weight is another method to maintain your blood sugar levels. Losing 5 to 10 percent of your body weight can reduce high glucose levels. The right diet plan and aerobic exercises (or any other form of exercise) can help you lose weight in a healthy manner.

References

1. "Type 2 Diabetes," Mayo Clinic, January 9, 2019.

2. "Type 1 Diabetes," Mayo Clinic, August 7, 2017.

3   "Double Diabetes," Diabetes.co.uk, March 25, 2011.

4. Thompson, Dennis. "'Double Diabetes' a New Threat," MedicineNet, October 31, 2016.

5. "Type 1 Diabetes in Children," Mayo Clinic, August 16, 2017.

Chapter 9

Gestational Diabetes and Diabetes-Related Women's Concerns

What Is Gestational Diabetes?

Gestational diabetes is a type of diabetes that is first seen in a pregnant woman who did not have diabetes before she was pregnant. Some women have more than one pregnancy affected by gestational diabetes. Gestational diabetes usually shows up in the middle of pregnancy. Doctors most often test for it between 24 and 28 weeks of pregnancy.

Often, gestational diabetes can be controlled through eating healthy foods and regular exercise. Sometimes, a woman with gestational diabetes must also take insulin.

Problems of Gestational Diabetes in Pregnancy

Blood sugar that is not well controlled in a woman with gestational diabetes can lead to problems for the pregnant woman and the fetus.

A Large Baby

Diabetes that is not well-controlled causes the baby's blood sugar to be high. The baby is "overfed" and is large for gestational age (LGA). Besides causing discomfort to the woman during the last few months of pregnancy, an LGA baby can lead to problems during delivery for both the mother and the baby. The mother might need a C-Section to deliver the baby. The baby can be born with nerve damage due to pressure on the shoulder during delivery.

About This Chapter: Text beginning with the heading "What Is Gestational Diabetes?" is excerpted from "Gestational Diabetes and Pregnancy," Centers for Disease Control and Prevention (CDC), June 2018; Text beginning with the heading "Diabetes and Women" is excerpted from "Diabetes and Women," Centers for Disease Control and Prevention (CDC), April 16, 2018.

Cesarean Section

A cesarean section (C-section) is an operation to deliver the baby through the mother's belly. A woman who has diabetes that is not well controlled has a higher chance of needing a C-section to deliver the baby. When the baby is delivered by a C-section, it takes longer for the woman to recover from childbirth.

High Blood Pressure

When a pregnant woman has high blood pressure, protein in her urine, and swelling in fingers and toes that does not go away, she might have preeclampsia. It is a serious problem that needs to be watched closely and managed by her doctor. High blood pressure can cause harm to both the woman and the fetus. It might lead to the baby being born early and also could cause seizures or a stroke (a blood clot or a bleed in the brain that can lead to brain damage) in the woman during labor and delivery. Women with diabetes have high blood pressure more often than women without diabetes.

Tips for Women with Gestational Diabetes

1. **Eat healthy foods.** Eat healthy foods from a meal plan made for a person with diabetes. A dietitian can help you create a healthy meal plan. A dietitian can also help you learn how to control your blood sugar while you are pregnant.

2. **Exercise regularly.** Exercise is another way to keep blood sugar under control. It helps to balance food intake. After checking with your doctor, you can exercise regularly during and after pregnancy. Get at least 30 minutes of moderate-intensity physical activity at least 5 days a week. This could be brisk walking, swimming, or actively playing with children.

3. **Monitor blood sugar often.** Because pregnancy causes the body's need for energy to change, blood sugar levels can change very quickly. Check your blood sugar often, as directed by your doctor.

4. **Take insulin, if needed.** Sometimes, a woman with gestational diabetes must take insulin. If insulin is ordered by your doctor, take it as directed in order to help keep blood sugar under control.

5. **Get tested for diabetes after pregnancy.** Get tested for diabetes 6 to 12 weeks after your baby is born, and then every 1 to 3 years. For most women with gestational diabetes, the diabetes goes away soon after delivery. When it does not go away, the diabetes is called "type 2 diabetes." Even if diabetes does go away after the baby is born, half of all women who had gestational diabetes develop type 2 diabetes later. It is important for a woman who has had gestational diabetes to continue to exercise and eat a healthy diet after pregnancy to prevent or delay getting type 2 diabetes. She should also remind her doctor to check her blood sugar every 1 to 3 years.

Low Blood Sugar

People with diabetes who take insulin or other diabetes medications can develop blood sugar that is too low. Low blood sugar can be very serious and even fatal, if not treated quickly. Seriously low blood sugar can be avoided if women watch their blood sugar closely and treat low blood sugar early.

If a woman's diabetes was not well-controlled during pregnancy, her baby can very quickly develop low blood sugar after birth. The baby's blood sugar must be watched for several hours after delivery.

Diabetes and Women

Women with diabetes have more to manage. Stay on track by checking your blood sugar often, eating healthy food, and being active so you can be your healthiest and feel your best.

Diabetes-Related Women's Concerns
Yeast and Urinary Tract Infections

Many women will get a vaginal yeast infection at some point, but women with diabetes are at a higher risk, especially if their blood sugar levels are high.

More than 50 percent of women will get a urinary tract infection (UTI) in their lifetime, and your risk may be higher if you have diabetes. Causes include high blood sugar levels and poor circulation (which reduces your body's ability to fight infections). Also, some women have bladders that do not empty all the way because of diabetes, creating a perfect environment for bacteria to grow.

How Is Diabetes Different for Women than It Is for Men?

Diabetes increases the risk of heart disease (the most common diabetes complication) by about four times in women but only about two times in men, and women have worse outcomes after a heart attack. Women are also at a higher risk of other diabetes-related complications, such as blindness, kidney disease, and depression.

Not only is diabetes different for women, it is different among women—African American, Hispanic/Latinx, American Indian/Alaska Native, and Asian/Pacific Islander women are more likely to have diabetes than White women.

How you manage diabetes may need to change over time depending on what is happening in your life. Here is what to expect and what you can do to stay on track.

53

What You Can Do: To prevent yeast infections and UTIs, keep your blood sugar levels as close to your target range as possible. Other ways to prevent UTIs include drinking a lot of water, wearing cotton underwear, and urinating often instead of waiting until your bladder is full.

Menstrual Cycle

Changes in hormone levels right before and during your period can make blood sugar levels hard to predict. You may also have longer or heavier periods, and food cravings can make managing diabetes harder. You may notice a pattern over time, or you may find that every period is different.

What You Can Do: Check your blood sugar often, and keep track of the results to see if there is a pattern. If you use insulin, you might need to take more in the days before your period. Talk to your doctor about changing your dosage if needed. Being active on most days, eating healthy food in the right amounts, and getting enough sleep can all help too.

Sex

Diabetes can lower your interest in sex and your ability to enjoy it. For some women, vaginal dryness can make intercourse uncomfortable or even painful. Causes can include nerve damage; reduced blood flow; medications; and hormonal changes, including those during pregnancy or menopause.

What You Can Do: Be sure to talk to your doctor if you are having any sexual issues. She or he can let you know your options, from using vaginal lubricants to doing exercises that can increase sexual response.

Birth Control

It is important to use birth control if you do not want to become pregnant or if you want to wait until your blood sugar levels are in your target range, since high blood sugar can cause problems during pregnancy for you and the fetus. There are many types of birth control methods, including intrauterine devices (IUDs); implants, injections; pills; patches; vaginal rings; and barrier methods, such as condoms and diaphragms. Choosing the right option for you will depend on whether you have any other medical conditions, current medicines you take, and other factors.

What You Can Do: Talk with your doctor about all your birth control options and risks. Continue checking your blood sugar, track the results, and let your doctor know if your levels go up.

Getting Pregnant

If you know you want to have a baby, planning ahead is really important. Diabetes can make it harder to get pregnant, and high blood sugar can increase your risk for:

- Preeclampsia (high blood pressure)

- Delivery by cesarean section (C-section)

- Miscarriage or stillbirth

The fetus's organs form during the first two months of pregnancy, and high blood sugar during that time can cause birth defects. High blood sugar during pregnancy can also increase the chance that your baby could:

- Be born too early

- Weight too much (making delivery harder)

- Have breathing problems or low blood sugar right after birth

What You Can Do: Work with your healthcare team to get your blood sugar levels in your target range and establish good habits, such as eating healthy and being active. Your blood sugar levels can change quickly, so check them often and adjust your food, activity, and medicine as needed with guidance from your doctor.

Chapter 10

Monogenic Forms of Diabetes

The most common forms of diabetes, type 1 and type 2, are polygenic, meaning they are related to a change, or defect, in multiple genes. Environmental factors, such as obesity in the case of type 2 diabetes, also play a part in the development of polygenic forms of diabetes. Polygenic forms of diabetes often run in families. Doctors diagnose polygenic forms of diabetes by testing blood glucose, also known as "blood sugar," in individuals with risk factors or symptoms of diabetes.

Genes provide the instructions for making proteins within the cell. If a gene has a change or mutation, the protein may not function properly. Genetic mutations that cause diabetes affect proteins that play a role in the ability of the body to produce insulin or in the ability of insulin to lower blood glucose. People typically have two copies of most genes, with one gene inherited from each parent.

What Are Monogenic Forms of Diabetes?

Some rare forms of diabetes result from mutations or changes in a single gene and are called "monogenic." In the United States, monogenic forms of diabetes account for about one to four percent of all cases of diabetes. In most cases of monogenic diabetes, the gene mutation is inherited from one or both parents. Sometimes, the gene mutation develops spontaneously, meaning that the mutation is not carried by either of the parents. Most mutations that cause monogenic diabetes reduce the body's ability to produce insulin, a protein produced in the pancreas that helps the body use glucose for energy.

About This Chapter: This chapter includes text excerpted from "Monogenic Diabetes (Neonatal Diabetes Mellitus and MODY)," National Institute of Diabetes and Digestive and Kidney Diseases (NIDDK), November 2017.

Neonatal diabetes mellitus (NDM) and maturity-onset diabetes of the young (MODY) are the two main forms of monogenic diabetes. NDM occurs in newborns and young infants. MODY is much more common than NDM and usually first occurs in adolescence or early adulthood.

Most cases of monogenic diabetes are incorrectly diagnosed. For example, when high blood glucose is first detected in adulthood, type 2 diabetes is often diagnosed instead of monogenic diabetes. If your healthcare provider thinks you might have monogenic diabetes, genetic testing may be needed to diagnose it and to identify which type. Testing of other family members may also be indicated to determine whether they are at risk for or already have a monogenic form of diabetes that is passed down from generation to generation. Some monogenic forms of diabetes can be treated with oral diabetes medicines (pills), while other forms require insulin injections. A correct diagnosis allows for proper treatment and can lead to better glucose control and improved health in the long term.

What Is Neonatal Diabetes Mellitus?

Neonatal diabetes mellitus is a monogenic form of diabetes that occurs in the first 6 to 12 months of life. NDM is a rare condition, accounting for up to 1 in 400,000 infants in the United States. Infants with NDM do not produce enough insulin, leading to an increase in blood glucose. NDM is often mistaken for type 1 diabetes, but type 1 diabetes is very rarely seen before 6 months of age. Diabetes that occurs in the first 6 months of life almost always has a genetic cause. Researchers have identified a number of specific genes and mutations that can cause NDM. In about half of those with NDM, the condition is lifelong and is called "permanent neonatal diabetes mellitus" (PNDM). In the rest of those with NDM, the condition is transient, or temporary, and disappears during infancy but can reappear later in life. This type of NDM is called "transient neonatal diabetes mellitus" (TNDM).

Clinical features of neonatal diabetes mellitus depend on the gene mutations a person has. Signs of NDM include frequent urination, rapid breathing, and dehydration. NDM can be diagnosed by finding elevated levels of glucose in blood or urine. The lack of insulin may cause the body to produce chemicals called "ketones," resulting in a potentially life-threatening condition called "diabetic ketoacidosis." Most fetuses with NDM do not grow well in the womb, and newborns with NDM are much smaller than those of the same gestational age, a condition called "intrauterine growth restriction." After birth, some infants fail to gain weight and grow as rapidly as other infants of the same age and sex. Appropriate therapy may improve and normalize growth and development.

What Is Maturity-Onset Diabetes of the Young?

Maturity-onset diabetes of the young is a monogenic form of diabetes that usually first occurs during adolescence or early adulthood. MODY accounts for up to 2 percent of all cases of diabetes in the United States in people 20 years of age and younger.

A number of different gene mutations have been shown to cause MODY, all of which limit the ability of the pancreas to produce insulin. This leads to high blood glucose levels and, in time, may damage body tissues, particularly tissues of the eyes, kidneys, nerves, and blood vessels.

Clinical features of MODY depend on the gene mutations a person has. People with certain types of mutations may have slightly high blood sugar levels that remain stable throughout life, have mild or no symptoms of diabetes, and do not develop any long-term complications. Their high blood glucose levels may only be discovered during routine blood tests. However, other mutations require specific treatment with either insulin or a type of oral diabetes medication called "sulfonylureas."

Maturity-onset diabetes of the young may be confused with type 1 or type 2 diabetes. In the past, people with MODY have generally not been overweight or obese, or have other risk factors for type 2 diabetes, such as high blood pressure or abnormal blood fat levels. However, as more people in the United States become overweight or obese, people with MODY may also be overweight or obese.

Although both type 2 diabetes and MODY can run in families, people with MODY typically have a family history of diabetes in multiple successive generations, meaning MODY is present in a grandparent, a parent, and a child.

How Is Monogenic Diabetes Diagnosed?

Genetic testing can diagnose most forms of monogenic diabetes. A correct diagnosis with proper treatment should lead to better glucose control and improved health in the long term.

Genetic testing is recommended if:

- Diabetes is diagnosed within the first six months of age.

- Diabetes is diagnosed in children and young adults, particularly those with a strong family history of diabetes, who do not have typical features of type 1 or type 2 diabetes, such as the presence of diabetes-related autoantibodies, obesity, and other metabolic features.

- A person has stable, mild fasting hyperglycemia, especially if obesity is not present.

What Do I Need to Know about Genetic Testing and Counseling?

Genetic testing for monogenic diabetes involves providing a blood or saliva sample from which deoxyribonucleic acid (DNA) is isolated. The DNA is analyzed for changes in the genes that cause monogenic diabetes. Genetic testing is done by specialized labs.

Abnormal results can determine the gene responsible for diabetes in a particular individual or show whether someone is likely to develop a monogenic form of diabetes in the future. Genetic testing can be helpful in selecting the most appropriate treatment for individuals with monogenic diabetes. Testing is also important in planning for pregnancy and to understand the risk of having a child with monogenic diabetes if you, your partner, or your family members have monogenic diabetes.

Most forms of neonatal diabetes mellitus and maturity-onset diabetes of the young are caused by autosomal dominant mutations, meaning that the condition can be passed on to children when only 1 parent carries or has the disease gene. With dominant mutations, a parent who carries the gene has a 50 percent chance of having an affected child with monogenic diabetes.

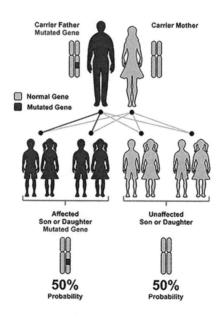

Figure 10.1. Autosomal Dominant

In most forms of MODY, a parent with MODY has a 50 percent chance of having a child with the disease.

In contrast, with the autosomal recessive disease, a mutation must be inherited from both parents. In this instance, a child has a 25 percent chance of having monogenic diabetes.

For recessive forms of monogenic diabetes, testing can indicate whether parents or siblings without disease are carriers for recessive genetic conditions that could be inherited by their children.

While not as common, it is possible to inherit mutations from the mother only. Also not as common are mutations that occur spontaneously.

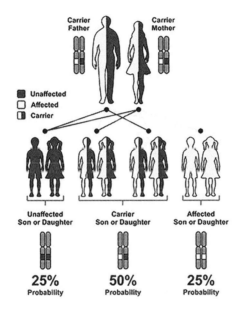

Figure 10.2. Autosomal Recessive

When both parents carry autosomal recessive mutations, a child has a 25 percent chance of having (or being affected by) the disease.

More information about the genes that cause NDM and MODY, the types of mutations responsible for the disease (autosomal dominant, autosomal recessive, X-linked, etc.), and clinical features is provided in the American Diabetes Association's (ADA) Standards of Medical Care in Diabetes.

If you suspect that you or a member of your family may have a monogenic form of diabetes, you should seek help from healthcare professionals—physicians and genetic counselors—who have specialized knowledge and experience in this area. They can determine whether genetic testing is appropriate; select the genetic tests that should be performed; and provide information about the basic principles of genetics, genetic testing options, and confidentiality issues. They also can review the test results with the patient or parent after testing, make recommendations about how to proceed, and discuss testing options for other family members.

How Is Monogenic Diabetes Treated and Managed?

Treatment varies depending on the specific genetic mutation that has caused a person's monogenic diabetes. People with certain forms of MODY and NDM can be treated with a sulfonylurea, an oral diabetes medicine that helps the body release more insulin into the blood. Other people may need insulin injections. Some people with MODY may not need medications and are able to manage their diabetes with lifestyle changes alone, which include physical activity and healthy food choices. Your physician and diabetes care team will work with you to develop a plan to treat and manage your diabetes based on the results of genetic testing.

Chapter 11

Diabetes Myths

Diabetes is a complex disease. You may have heard conflicting theories on what causes it, how it is diagnosed, and how it is managed. If you are affected by diabetes, you will want the truth about the disease. Here are some common myths that you may have heard:

There is no diabetes in my family, so I do not have to worry. Diabetes does run in families, but many people diagnosed with the disease have no close family members who have it. Lifestyle, heredity, and possibly other factors, such as certain viruses, may increase risk for the disease.

It is called "sugar diabetes," so it must come from the sugar I eat. When you eat food, the body turns it into a form of energy called "glucose," also known as "blood sugar." Glucose is not the refined sugar that you buy in stores. Insulin helps move the blood sugar into the body's cells for energy. When the body's own insulin does not work well or when not enough is made, the blood sugar level rises. Then the person has diabetes.

I'll know that I have diabetes by my symptoms. A person with type 1 diabetes, usually seen in children and young adults, will have obvious symptoms, because they have little or no insulin, the hormone that controls the blood sugar level. However, people with type 2 diabetes, which usually occurs later in life, or women who have gestational diabetes, the diabetes that only appears during pregnancy, may have few or no symptoms. Their symptoms are milder since they still produce some insulin. Unfortunately, they do not make enough insulin, or it is not being used properly. Only a blood test can tell for sure if someone has diabetes.

About This Chapter: This chapter includes text excerpted from "Diabetes Myths," Centers for Disease Control and Prevention (CDC), June 2017.

My doctor says I have "borderline" diabetes. Since I have just a "touch of sugar," I do not have to worry. There is no such thing as borderline diabetes. To many people, "borderline" means they do not really have the disease, so they do not have to make any changes to control it. This is wrong. If you have diabetes, you have diabetes. Diabetes must be treated and taken seriously.

By drinking water, I can wash away the extra sugar in my blood and cure my diabetes. Although you can wash away sugar spilled on a table, you cannot wash away a high blood sugar level by drinking water. However, you can control diabetes by eating healthy food, being physically active, controlling your weight, seeing your medical team regularly, taking prescribed medications, and monitoring your blood sugar often.

Insulin is a cure for diabetes. Insulin is not a cure for diabetes. At this point, there is no cure; there are only medicine and behaviors that can control diabetes. Insulin helps to control diabetes by keeping the blood sugar from rising.

My friend takes insulin pills to control her diabetes. Insulin is a protein; it cannot be taken by mouth because the stomach would not digest it. Insulin must be given by injection or insulin pump through the skin. Diabetes pills help by making the body produce more insulin, use its own insulin better, produce less blood sugar from the liver, or limit carbohydrate absorption after a meal.

If I do not take diabetes medicine, my diabetes must not be serious. Not everyone who has diabetes takes diabetes medicine. If the body produces some insulin, weight loss, healthy eating habits, and regular physical activity can help insulin work more effectively. However, diabetes does change over time, and diabetes medicine may be needed later.

If I get diabetes, I will never be able to eat any sugar. To control one's blood sugar, all sources of carbohydrates must be controlled. Carbohydrates include starchy foods like pasta and bread as well as sugary foods like candy. Even juice, milk, and fruit all contain carbohydrates, so they must be eaten in moderate amounts. With careful planning, small amounts of sugar can replace other carbohydrates usually eaten at a meal. Too much sugar is bad for everyone. It provides only empty calories.

I have diabetes, and I've seen its effect on family members. I know there is nothing I can do about it. Remember that diabetes is serious, common, costly, and CONTROLLABLE. There are many things people with diabetes can do to live a full life, while preventing or delaying complications. You can control your diabetes by eating healthy foods, staying active, losing weight if needed, taking medicine as prescribed, testing your blood sugar, and seeing your healthcare team.

But... You Don't Look Like You Have Diabetes!

Has anyone ever said this to you? You might have wanted to reply "what do you think diabetes looks like?" Because the truth is you cannot tell if someone has it by looking at them. Diabetes can look like anyone:

- All ages: children, teens, young adults, and older adults
- All weights: underweight, normal weight, and overweight
- All fitness levels
- All races/ethnicities

(Source: "But You Don't Look Like You Have Diabetes," Centers for Disease Control and Prevention (CDC).)

Part Two
Medical Management of Diabetes

Chapter 12

You and Your Diabetes Care Team

A team approach to diabetes care can effectively help people cope with the vast array of complications that can arise from diabetes. People with diabetes can lower their risk for microvascular complications, such as eye disease and kidney disease; macrovascular complications, such as heart disease and stroke; and other diabetes complications, such as nerve damage, by:

- Controlling their ABCs (A1C, blood pressure, cholesterol, and smoking cessation)

- Following an individualized meal plan

- Engaging in regular physical activity

- Avoiding tobacco use

- Taking medicines as prescribed

- Coping effectively with the demands of a complex chronic disease

Patients who increase their use of effective behavioral interventions to lower the risk of diabetes—and treatments to improve glycemic control and cardiovascular risk profiles—can prevent or delay the progression of kidney failure, vision loss, nerve damage, lower extremity amputation, and cardiovascular disease. This, in turn, can lead to increased patient satisfaction with care, better quality of life, improved health outcomes, and ultimately, lower healthcare costs.

The challenge is to broaden the delivery of care by expanding the healthcare team to include several types of healthcare professionals. Collaborative teams vary according to patients' needs,

About This Chapter: This chapter includes text excerpted from "Team Care Approach for Diabetes Management," Centers for Disease Control and Prevention (CDC), June 15, 2011. Reviewed June 2019.

patient load, organizational constraints, resources, clinical setting, geographic location, and professional skills.

> **Patient Case Example**
>
> A dentist needs to schedule a patient for several procedures and asks about the timing of the patient's morning insulin. The patient is confused about this complicated medication regimen and asks, "Should I just skip all medicines that day until after you work on my teeth?" The dentist phones the patient's pharmacist to arrange a consultation. The pharmacist collaborates with the primary care clinician to develop an individualized medication schedule and advises the patient and dentist on medication usage on the day of the procedure.

Pharmacy, Podiatry, Optometry, and Dentistry and the Team Approach

You and other pharmacy, podiatry, optometry, and dentistry (PPOD) providers play an integral role in the team care approach to diabetes care. When you are educated about the complications of diabetes care issues in your own and other PPOD disciplines, you can better recognize symptomatic concerns that warrant a timely referral and reinforce annual screening recommendations that are proven to lower the risk of serious complications for diabetic patients. A multidisciplinary team approach is critical to success in diabetes care and complications prevention. Evidence indicates that a team approach:

- Can facilitate diabetes management

- Can lower the risk for chronic disease complications

- Helps educate about ways to reduce risk factors for type 2 diabetes in your patients' family members

Healthcare Team for People with Diabetes

There are many other possible members of the healthcare team in addition to physicians (e.g., primary care, endocrinologist, obstetrician-gynecologist, ophthalmologist). This team could include (but is not limited to):

- Pharmacists

- Podiatrists

- Optometrists

- Dental care professionals

- Primary care physicians

- Physician assistants

- Nurse practitioners

- Dietitians

- Certified diabetes educators

- Community health workers

- Mental health professionals

Other Valuable Team Members

Clinical care teams can be augmented by including the resources and support of community partners such as:

- School nurses

- Trained peer leaders

Nontraditional approaches to healthcare can expand access to team care and, if used effectively, can build team care practices. These approaches include telehealth, shared medical appointments, and group education. For instance, pharmacist-directed telehealth programs have improved outcomes in blood pressure and diabetes medication management. There are also opportunities to partner with primary care providers in shared group appointments (SGAs). These shared group visits allow time for learning and integration of new knowledge and skills. A literature review showed that SGAs build synergy between healthcare providers and patients, while using group interactions to increase knowledge and self-care skills. All of these team members play important roles in the delivery of care for people with diabetes. When you work together using a team care approach, you can:

- Minimize patients' health risks through assessment, intervention, and surveillance

- Identify problems early and initiate timely treatment

> ## Key Messages All Healthcare Providers Can Reinforce
> - Emphasize the importance of metabolic control and the control of other cardiovascular risk factors such as the ABCs.
> - Promote a healthy lifestyle that includes physical activity, healthful eating, and coping skills.
> - Explain the benefits of diabetes comprehensive team care.
> - Recommend routine checkups to prevent complications: a dental exam, a comprehensive foot exam, and a complete dilated eye exam.
> - Reinforce self-exams for foot care and dental care, and others as appropriate.
> - Recognize the danger signs for foot and dental problems and seek help from a healthcare provider.
> - Promote the pharmacist's role in drug therapy management.

Promoting Team Interaction

Below are some tools and resources you can use to promote interaction among PPOD professionals and other providers:

- The National Diabetes Education Program's (NDEP) redesigning the healthcare team illustrates how teams can work together effectively. Examples from the peer-reviewed literature and case studies that show the diversity and effectiveness of healthcare professional teams working with people who have diabetes include:

    - Community-based primary care providers who involve a pharmacist and dietitian in implementing treatment algorithms, nurse and dietitian case managers, and educators who help to improve patients' weight loss and A1C values

    - A nurse practitioner-physician team that manages patients with diabetes and hypertension

    - Healthcare professionals who use telehealth to improve eye care, nutrition counseling, and diabetes self-management education

    - Pharmacists who work with company employees who have diabetes and their physicians to improve clinical measures and lower healthcare costs

    - Trained community health workers who bridge the gap among traditional healthcare teams to improve access to diabetes healthcare, complications assessment, and education in underserved communities

- Podiatrists and other healthcare professionals who help reduce lower-extremity amputation rates in foot care clinics

- Dental and eye care professionals who help prevent and manage diabetes complications

- The NDEP's comprehensive *Diabetes Head to Toe Checklist Examination Report* was developed by the NDEP Healthcare Providers Stakeholders' Group (comprises of physicians, nurses, physician assistants, and diabetes educators), and the PPOD Providers Stakeholders' Group (comprised of providers in all four of the PPOD fields—pharmacy, podiatry, optometry, and dentistry)—to foster collaboration. The groups developed the checklist to support coordination of care and to recognize the following variables:

  - Coordination will help ensure that patients understand and can implement the intended treatment plan and can identify drug and disease management and psychosocial problems in a timely manner.

  - Coordination of care presents many challenges when delivered by multiple providers in a variety of settings.

  - PPOD professionals are often a primary point of care for people with type 2 diabetes. They have an important role in ensuring that diabetes care is continuous and patient-centered.

The checklist was pilot-tested by a range of healthcare providers and was found to be useful in a real-world clinical setting. They indicated that they were likely to change their practice to more of a team approach, incorporating the members of the team, or to adopt a referral approach. The providers also reported that the checklist helped them educate their patients about how preventive care can decrease the risk of diabetes complications. Further, 30 percent indicated that the checklist has useful application in electronic medical record/electronic health record systems.

Chapter 13

Steps to Manage Your Diabetes for Life

> You can manage your diabetes and live a long and healthy life by taking care of yourself each day.
>
> Diabetes can affect almost every part of your body. Therefore, you will need to manage your blood glucose levels, also called blood sugar. Managing your blood glucose, as well as your blood pressure and cholesterol, can help prevent the health problems that can occur when you have diabetes.
>
> *(Source: "Managing Diabetes," National Institute of Diabetes and Digestive and Kidney Diseases (NIDDK).)*

Step 1: Learn about Diabetes
What Is Diabetes?

There are three main types of diabetes:

- **Type 1 diabetes**—Your body does not make insulin. This is a problem because you need insulin to take the sugar (glucose) from the foods you eat and turn it into energy for your body. You need to take insulin every day to live.

- **Type 2 diabetes**—Your body does not make or use insulin well. You may need to take pills or insulin to help control your diabetes. Type 2 is the most common type of diabetes.

About This Chapter: This chapter includes text excerpted from "4 Steps to Manage Your Diabetes for Life," National Institute of Diabetes and Digestive and Kidney Diseases (NIDDK), January 2016.

- **Gestational diabetes**—Some women get this kind of diabetes when they are pregnant. Most of the time, it goes away after the baby is born. But, even if it goes away, these women and their children have a greater chance of getting diabetes later in life.

You are the most important member of your healthcare team.

You are the one who manages your diabetes day by day. Talk to your doctor about how you can best care for your diabetes to stay healthy. Some other healthcare professionals who can help are:

- Dentist
- Diabetes doctor
- Diabetes educator
- Dietitian
- Eye doctor
- Foot doctor
- Friends and family
- Mental-health counselor
- Nurse
- Nurse practitioner
- Pharmacist
- Social worker

How to Learn More about Diabetes

- Take classes to learn more about living with diabetes. To find a class, check with your healthcare team, hospital, or area health clinic. You can also search online.

- Join a support group—in-person or online—to get peer support with managing your diabetes.

Take Diabetes Seriously

You may have heard people say they have "a touch of diabetes" or that their "sugar is a little high." These words suggest that diabetes is not a serious disease. That is not correct. Diabetes is serious, but you can learn to manage it.

People with diabetes need to make healthy food choices, stay at a healthy weight, move more every day, and take their medicine even when they feel good. It is a lot to do. It is not easy, but it is worth it.

Why Take Care of Your Diabetes?

Taking care of yourself and your diabetes can help you feel good today and in the future. When your blood sugar is close to normal, you are likely to:

- Have more energy

- Be less tired and thirsty

- Need to urinate less often

- Heal better

- Have fewer skin or bladder infections

You will also have less chance of having health problems caused by diabetes, such as:

- Heart attack or stroke

- Eye problems that can lead to trouble seeing or going blind

- Pain, tingling, or numbness in your hands and feet, also called "nerve damage"

- Kidney problems that can cause your kidneys to stop working

- Teeth and gum problems

Actions You Can Take

- Ask your healthcare team what type of diabetes you have.

- Learn where you can go for support.

- Learn how caring for your diabetes helps you feel good today and in the future.

Step 2: Know Your Diabetes ABCs

Talk to your healthcare team about how to manage your A1C, blood pressure, and cholesterol. This can help lower your chances of having a heart attack, stroke, or other diabetes problems.

A for the A1C Test
What Is It?

The A1C is a blood test that measures your average blood sugar level over the past three months. It is different from the blood sugar checks you do each day.

Why Is It Important?

You need to know your blood sugar levels over time. You do not want those numbers to get too high. High levels of blood sugar can harm your heart, blood vessels, kidneys, feet, and eyes.

What Is the A1C Goal?

The A1C goal for many people with diabetes is below seven. It may be different for you. Ask what your goal should be.

B for Blood Pressure
What Is It?

Blood pressure is the force of your blood against the wall of your blood vessels.

Why Is It Important?

If your blood pressure gets too high, it makes your heart work too hard. It can cause a heart attack, stroke, and damage your kidneys and eyes.

What Is the Blood Pressure Goal?

The blood pressure goal for most people with diabetes is below 140/90. It may be different for you. Ask what your goal should be.

C for Cholesterol
What Is It?

There are two kinds of cholesterol in your blood: low-density lipoproteins (LDL) and high-density lipoproteins (HDL).

LDL or "bad" cholesterol can build up and clog your blood vessels. It can cause a heart attack or stroke.

HDL or "good" cholesterol helps remove the "bad" cholesterol from your blood vessels.

What Are the Low-Density Lipoproteins and High-Density Lipoproteins Goals?

Ask what your cholesterol numbers should be. Your goals may be different from other people. If you are over 40 years of age, you may need to take a statin drug for heart health.

Actions You Can Take

Ask your healthcare team what your A1C, blood pressure, and cholesterol numbers are and what they should be. Your ABC goals will depend on how long you have had diabetes, other health problems, and how hard your diabetes is to manage.

Step 3: Learn How to Live with Diabetes

It is common to feel overwhelmed, sad, or angry when you are living with diabetes. You may know the steps you should take to stay healthy but have trouble sticking with your plan over time. This section has tips on how to cope with your diabetes, eat well, and be active.

Cope with Your Diabetes

- Stress can raise your blood sugar. Learn ways to lower your stress. Try deep breathing, gardening, taking a walk, meditating, working on your hobby, or listening to your favorite music.

- Ask for help if you feel down. A mental-health counselor, support group, member of the clergy, friend, or family member who will listen to your concerns may help you feel better.

Eat Well

- Make a diabetes meal plan with help from your healthcare team.
- Choose foods that are lower in calories, saturated fat, trans fat, sugar, and salt.
- Eat foods with more fiber, such as whole grain cereals, breads, crackers, rice, or pasta.
- Choose foods such as fruits, vegetables, whole grains, bread and cereals, and low-fat or skim milk and cheese.

- Drink water instead of juice and regular soda.

- When eating a meal, fill half of your plate with fruits and vegetables; one quarter with a lean protein, such as beans, or chicken or turkey without the skin; and one quarter with a whole grain, such as brown rice or whole wheat pasta.

Be Active

- Set a goal to be more active most days of the week. Start slowly by taking 10-minute walks, 3 times a day.

- Twice a week, work to increase your muscle strength. Use stretch bands, participate in yoga*, do heavy gardening (digging and planting with tools), or try push-ups.

- Stay at or get to a healthy weight by using your meal plan and moving more.

A mind and body practice with origins in ancient Indian philosophy.

Know What to Do Every Day

- Take your medicines for diabetes and any other health problems even when you feel good. Ask your doctor if you need aspirin to prevent a heart attack or stroke. Tell your doctor if you cannot afford your medicines or if you have any side effects.

- Check your feet every day for cuts, blisters, red spots, and swelling. Call your healthcare team right away about any sores that do not go away.

- Brush your teeth and floss every day to keep your mouth, teeth, and gums healthy.

- Stop smoking.

- Keep track of your blood sugar. You may want to check it one or more times a day. Keep a record of your blood sugar numbers, and be sure to talk about it with your healthcare team.

- Check your blood pressure if your doctor advises and keep a record of it.

Talk to Your Healthcare Team

- Ask your doctor if you have any questions about your diabetes.

- Report any changes in your health.

Actions You Can Take

- Ask for a healthy meal plan.

- Ask about ways to be more active.

- Ask how and when to test your blood sugar and how to use the results to manage your diabetes.

- Use these tips to help with your self-care.

- Discuss how your diabetes plan is working for you each time you visit your healthcare team.

Step 4: Get Routine Care to Stay Healthy

See your healthcare team at least twice a year to find and treat any problems early.

At each visit, be sure you have a:

- Blood pressure check

- Foot check

- Weight check

- Review of your self-care plan

Two times each year, have an:

- A1C test. It may be checked more often if it is over seven.

Once each year, be sure you have a:

- Cholesterol test

- Complete foot exam

- Dental exam to check teeth and gums

- Dilated eye exam to check for eye problems

- Flu shot

- Urine and a blood test to check for kidney problems

At least once in your lifetime, get a:

- Pneumonia shot

- Hepatitis B shot

Medicare and Diabetes

If you have Medicare, check to see how your plan covers diabetes care. Medicare covers some of the costs for:

- Diabetes education
- Diabetes supplies
- Diabetes medicine
- Visits with a dietitian
- Special shoes, if you need them

Actions You Can Take

- Ask your healthcare team about these and other tests you may need. Ask what your results mean.
- Write down the date and time of your next visit.

If you have Medicare, check your plan.

Chapter 14

Know Your Blood Sugar Numbers

Checking your blood sugar, also called "blood glucose," is an important part of diabetes care. This chapter tells you:

- Why it helps you to know your blood sugar numbers

- How to check your blood sugar levels

- What are target blood sugar levels

- What to do if your levels are too low or too high

- How to pay for these tests

Why Do I Need to Know My Blood Sugar Numbers?

Your blood sugar numbers show how well your diabetes is managed. And, managing your diabetes means that you have a lesser chance of having serious health problems, such as kidney disease and vision loss.

As you check your blood sugar, you can see what makes your numbers go up and down. For example, you may see that when you are stressed or eat certain foods, your numbers go up. And, you may see that when you take your medicine and are active, your numbers go down. This information lets you know what is working for you and what needs to change.

About This Chapter: This chapter includes text excerpted from "Know Your Blood Sugar Numbers: Use Them to Manage Your Diabetes," National Institute of Diabetes and Digestive and Kidney Diseases (NIDDK), March 2016.

How Is Blood Sugar Measured?

There are two ways to measure blood sugar.

- Blood sugar checks that you do yourself. These tell you what your blood sugar level is at the time you test.

- The A1C is a test done in a lab or at your provider's office. This test tells you your average blood sugar level over the past two to three months.

How Do I Check My Blood Sugar?

You use a blood glucose meter to check your blood sugar. This device uses a small drop of blood from your finger to measure your blood sugar level. You can get the meter and supplies in a drugstore or by mail.

Read the directions that come with your meter to learn how to check your blood sugar. Your healthcare team also can show you how to use your meter. Write the date, time, and result of the test in your blood sugar record. Take your blood sugar record and meter to each visit and talk about your results with your healthcare team.

What Are Target Blood Sugar Levels for People with Diabetes?

A target is something that you aim for or try to reach. Your healthcare team may also use the term goal. People with diabetes have blood sugar targets that they try to reach at different times of the day. These targets are:

- Right before your meal: 80 to 130

- Two hours after the start of the meal: below 180

Talk with your healthcare team about what blood sugar numbers are right for you.

How Often Should I Check My Blood Sugar?

The number of times that you check your blood sugar will depend on the type of diabetes that you have and the type of medicine you take to treat your diabetes. For example, people who take insulin may need to check more often than people who do not take insulin. Talk with your healthcare team about how often to check your blood sugar.

The common times for checking your blood sugar are when you first wake up (fasting), before a meal, two hours after a meal, and at bedtime. Talk with your healthcare team about what times are best for you to check your blood sugar.

What Should I Do If My Blood Sugar Gets Too High?

High blood sugar is also called "hyperglycemia." It means that your blood sugar level is higher than your target level or over 180. Having high blood sugar levels over time can lead to long-term, serious health problems.

If you feel very tired, thirsty, have blurry vision, or need to pee more often, your blood sugar may be high.

Check your blood sugar and see if it is above your target level or over 180. If it is too high, one way to lower it is to drink a large glass of water and exercise by taking a brisk walk. Call your healthcare team if your blood sugar is high more than 3 times in 2 weeks and you do not know why.

What Should I Do If My Blood Sugar Gets Too Low?

Low blood sugar is also called "hypoglycemia." It means your blood sugar level drops below 70. Having low blood sugar is dangerous and needs to be treated right away. Anyone with diabetes can have low blood sugar. You have a greater chance of having low blood sugar if you take insulin or certain pills for diabetes.

Carry supplies for treating low blood sugar with you. If you feel shaky, sweaty, or very hungry, check your blood sugar. Even if you feel none of these things but think you may have low blood sugar, check it.

If your meter shows that your blood sugar is lower than 70, do one of the following things right away:

- Chew 4 glucose tablets.
- Drink 4 ounces of fruit juice.
- Drink 4 ounces of regular soda, not diet soda.
- Chew 4 pieces of hard candy.

After taking one of these treatments, wait for 15 minutes, then check your blood sugar again. Repeat these steps until your blood sugar is 70 or above. After your blood sugar gets back up to 70 or more, eat a snack if your next meal is one hour or more away.

If you often have low blood sugar, check your blood sugar before driving and treat it if it is low.

What Do I Need to Know about the A1C Test?

The A1C test tells you and your healthcare team your average blood sugar level over the past two to three months. It also helps you and your team decide the type and amount of diabetes medicine you need.

What Is a Good A1C Goal for You?

For many people with diabetes, the A1C goal is below seven. This number is different from the blood sugar numbers that you check each day. You and your healthcare team will decide on an A1C goal that is right for you.

How Often Do I Need an A1C Test?

You need to get an A1C test at least two times a year. You need it more often if:

- Your number is higher than your goal number
- Your diabetes treatment changes

How Do I Pay for These Tests and Supplies?

Medicaid and most private insurance plans pay for the A1C test and some of the cost of supplies for checking your blood sugar. Check your plan or ask your healthcare team for help finding a low cost or free supplies. Ask your healthcare team what to do if you run out of test strips.

What If I Have Trouble Getting to My Blood Sugar Goals?

There may be times when you have trouble reaching your blood sugar goals. This does not mean that you have failed. It means that you and your healthcare team should see if changes are needed. Call your healthcare team if your blood sugar is often too high or too low. Taking action will help you be healthy today and in the future.

Story of John

At each visit, John and his healthcare team look at his A1C test results, his blood glucose meter and his blood sugar record to see if his treatment is working. At today's visit, John's A1C and blood sugar numbers are too high. John and his healthcare team talk about what he can do to get closer to his A1C and blood sugar goals. John decides he will be more active. He will:

- Increase his walking time to 30 minutes every day after dinner.
- Check his fasting blood sugar in the morning to see if being more active improves his blood sugar.
- Call his doctor in 1 month for a change in medicine if his blood sugar levels are still too high.
- Have his A1C tested again in 3 months to see if his new plan is working.

Things to Remember

- Check your blood sugar as many times a day as your healthcare team suggests.
- Have your A1C checked at least 2 times a year.
- Keep a record of your blood sugar and A1C numbers.
- Take your blood glucose meter and blood sugar record to your visit and show them to your healthcare team. Tell your healthcare team how you think you are doing.
- Call your healthcare team if your blood sugar is often too high or too low.

Chapter 15

Blood Glucose Monitoring

What Does Blood Glucose Monitoring Test Do?

This is a test system for use at home or in healthcare settings to measure the amount of sugar (glucose) in your blood.

What Is Glucose?

Glucose is a sugar that your body uses as a source of energy. Unless you have diabetes, your body regulates the amount of glucose in your blood. People with diabetes may need special diets and medications to control blood glucose.

What Type of Test Is This?

This is a quantitative test, which means that you will find out the amount of glucose present in your blood sample.

Why Should You Take This Test?

You should take this test if you have diabetes, and you need to monitor your blood sugar (glucose) levels. You and your doctor can use the results to:

- Determine your daily adjustments in treatment

About This Chapter: Text beginning with the heading "What Does Blood Glucose Monitoring Test Do?" is excerpted from "Blood Glucose Monitoring Devices," U.S. Food and Drug Administration (FDA), April 4, 2019; Text under the heading "Continuous Glucose Monitoring?" is excerpted from "Continuous Glucose Monitoring," National Institute of Diabetes and Digestive and Kidney Diseases (NIDDK), June 2017.

- Know if you have dangerously high or low levels of glucose

- Understand how your diet and exercise change your glucose levels

The Diabetes Control and Complications Trial (DCCT) (1993) showed that good glucose control using home monitors led to fewer disease complications.

How Often Should You Test Your Glucose?

Follow your doctor's recommendations about how often you should test your glucose. You may need to test yourself several times each day to determine adjustments in your diet or treatment.

Maintaining Your Blood Glucose Meter

- Keep your meter clean.
- Test your meter regularly with control solution.
- Keep extra batteries charged and ready.
- Store your meter and supplies properly. Heat and humidity can damage test strips.
- Replace the bottle cap promptly after removing a test strip.

(Source: "Home Healthcare Medical Devices: Blood Glucose Meters," U.S. Food and Drug Administration (FDA).)

What Should Your Glucose Levels Be?

According to the American Diabetes Association (Standards of Medical Care in Diabetes—2017. Diabetes Care, January 2017, vol. 40, Supplement 1, S11-S24) the blood glucose levels for an adult without diabetes are below 100 mg/dL before meals and fasting, and are less than 140 mg/dL 2 hours after meals.

People with diabetes should consult their doctor or healthcare provider to set appropriate blood glucose goals. You should treat your low or high blood glucose as recommended by your healthcare provider.

The accuracy of this test depends on many factors including:

- The quality of your meter

- The quality of your test strips

    - Always use new test strips that are authorized for sale in the United States. The U.S. Food and Drug Administration (FDA) has issued a safety communication warning about the risks of using previously owned test strips or test strips that are not authorized for sale in the United States.

- How well you perform the test. For example, you should wash and dry your hands before testing and closely follow the instructions for operating your meter.

- Your hematocrit (the amount of red blood cells in the blood). If you are severely dehydrated or anemic, your test results may be less accurate. Your healthcare provider can tell you if your hematocrit is low or high, and they can discuss with you how it may affect your glucose testing.

- Interfering substances. Some substances, such as vitamin C, Tylenol, and uric acid, may interfere with your glucose testing. Check the instructions for your meter and test strips to find out what substances may affect the testing accuracy.

- Altitude, temperature, and humidity. A high altitude, low and high temperatures, and humidity can cause unpredictable effects on glucose results. Check the meter manual and test strip package insert for more information.

- Store and handle the meter and strips according to the manufacturer's instructions. It is important to store test strip vials closed

How Do You Take This Test?

Before you test your blood glucose, you must read and understand the instructions for your meter. In general, you prick your finger with a lancet to get a drop of blood. Then you place the blood on a disposable test strip that is inserted in your meter. The test strip contains chemicals that react with glucose. Some meters measure the amount of electricity that passes through the test strip. Others measure how much light reflects from it. In the United States, meters report results in milligrams of glucose per deciliter of blood, or mg/dl.

You can get information about your meter and test strips from several different sources, including the toll-free number in the manual that comes with your meter or on the manufacturer's website. If you have an urgent problem, always contact your healthcare provider or a local emergency room for advice.

How Do You Choose a Glucose Meter?

There are many different types of meters available for purchase that differ in several ways, including:

- Accuracy

- Amount of blood needed for each test
- How easy it is to use
- Pain associated with using the product
- Testing speed
- Overall size
- Ability to store test results in memory
- Likelihood of interferences
- Ability to transmit data to a computer
- Cost of the meter
- Cost of the test strips used
- Doctor's recommendation
- Technical support provided by the manufacturer
- Special features, such as automatic timing, error codes, a large display screen, or spoken instructions or results

Talk to your healthcare provider about the right glucose meter for you, and how to use it.

How Can You Check Your Meter's Performance?

There are three ways to make sure your meter works properly:

1. Use liquid control solutions:

    - Every time you open a new container of test strips
    - Occasionally as you use the container of test strips
    - If you drop the meter
    - Whenever you get unusual results

    To test a liquid control solution, you test a drop of these solutions just as you would test a drop of your blood. The value you get should match the value written on the test strip vial label.

2. Use electronic checks. Every time you turn on your meter, it does an electronic check. If it detects a problem, it will give you an error code. Look in your meter's manual to

see what the error codes mean and how to fix the problem. If you are unsure if your meter is working properly, call the toll-free number in your meter's manual, or contact your healthcare provider.

3. Compare your meter with a blood glucose test performed in a laboratory. Take your meter with you to your next appointment with your healthcare provider. Ask your provider to watch your testing technique to make sure you are using the meter correctly. Ask your healthcare provider to have your blood tested with a laboratory method. If the values you obtain on your glucose meter match the laboratory values, then your meter is working well and you are using good technique.

What Should You Do If Your Meter Malfunctions?

If your meter malfunctions, you should tell your healthcare provider and contact the company that made your meter and strips.

Alternative Site Testing

Some meters allow you to test blood from sites other than the fingertip. Examples of such alternative sampling sites are your palm, upper arm, forearm, thigh, or calf. Alternative site testing (AST) should not be performed at times when your blood glucose may be changing rapidly, as these alternative sampling sites may provide inaccurate results at those times. You should use only blood from your fingertip to test if any of the following applies:

- You have just taken insulin.
- You think your blood sugar is low.
- You are not aware of symptoms when you become hypoglycemic.
- The results do not agree with the way you feel.
- You have just eaten.
- You have just exercised.
- You are ill.
- You are under stress.

Also, you should never use results from an alternative sampling site to calibrate a continuous glucose monitor (CGM), or in insulin dosing calculations.

Continuous Glucose Monitoring

Continuous glucose monitoring automatically tracks blood glucose levels throughout the day and night. You can see your glucose level anytime at a glance. You can also review how your glucose changes over a few hours or days to see trends. Seeing glucose levels in real time can help you make more informed decisions throughout the day about how to balance your food, physical activity, and medicines.

How Does a Continuous Glucose Monitor Work?

A continuous glucose monitor works through a tiny sensor inserted under your skin, usually on your belly or arm. The sensor measures your interstitial glucose level, which is the glucose found in the fluid between the cells. The sensor tests glucose every few minutes. A transmitter wirelessly sends the information to a monitor.

The monitor may be part of an insulin pump or a separate device, which you might carry in a pocket or purse. Some CGMs send information directly to a smartphone or tablet.

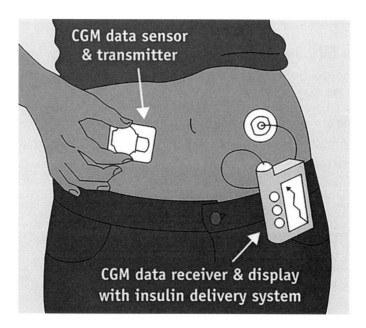

Figure 15.1. Continuous Glucose Monitor (CGM)

A tiny CGM sensor under the skin checks glucose. A transmitter sends data to a receiver. The CGM receiver may be part of an insulin pump, as shown here, or a separate device.

Special Features of a Continuous Glucose Monitoring

Continuous glucose monitors are always on and recording glucose levels—whether you are showering, working, exercising, or sleeping. Many CGMs have special features that work with information from your glucose readings:

- An alarm can sound when your glucose level goes too low or too high.

- You can note your meals, physical activity, and medicines in a CGM device too, alongside your glucose levels.

- You can download data to a computer or smart device to more easily see your glucose trends.

Some models can send information right away to a second person's smartphone—perhaps a parent, partner, or caregiver. For example, if a child's glucose drops dangerously low overnight, the CGM could be set to wake a parent in the next room.

Special Requirements Needed to Use a Continuous Glucose Monitoring

Twice a day, you may need to check the CGM itself. You will test a drop of blood on a standard glucose meter. The glucose reading should be similar on both devices.

You will also need to replace the CGM sensor every three to seven days, depending on the model.

For safety, it is important to take action when a CGM alarm sounds about high or low blood glucose. You should follow your treatment plan to bring your glucose into the target range, or get help.

Who Can Use a Continuous Glucose Monitoring?

Most people who use CGMs have type 1 diabetes. Research is underway to learn how CGMs might help people with type 2 diabetes.

Continuous glucose monitors are approved for use by adults and children with a doctor's prescription. Some models may be used for children as young as the age of two. Your doctor may recommend a CGM if you or your child:

- Are on intensive insulin therapy, also called "tight blood sugar control"

- Have hypoglycemia unawareness

- Often have high or low blood glucose

Your doctor may suggest using a CGM system all the time or only for a few days to help adjust your diabetes care plan.

What Are the Benefits of a Continuous Glucose Monitoring?

Compared with a standard blood glucose meter, using a CGM system can help you:

- Better manage your glucose levels every day

- Have fewer low blood glucose emergencies

- Need fewer finger sticks

A graphic on the CGM screen shows whether your glucose is rising or dropping—and how quickly—so you can choose the best way to reach your target glucose level.

Over time, good management of glucose greatly helps people with diabetes stay healthy and prevent complications of the disease. People who gain the largest benefit from a CGM are those who use it every day or nearly every day.

What Are the Limits of a Continuous Glucose Monitoring?

Researchers are working to make CGMs more accurate and easier to use. But, you still need a finger-stick glucose test twice a day to check the accuracy of your CGM against a standard blood glucose meter.

With most CGM models, you cannot yet rely on the CGM alone to make treatment decisions. For example, before changing your insulin dose, you must first confirm a CGM reading by doing a finger-stick glucose test.

A continuous glucose monitoring system is more expensive than using a standard glucose meter. Check with your health insurance plan or Medicare to see whether the costs will be covered.

Chapter 16

Glucose in Urine Test

What Is a Glucose in Urine Test?

A glucose in urine test measures the amount of glucose in your urine. Glucose is a type of sugar. It is your body's main source of energy. A hormone called "insulin" helps move glucose from your bloodstream into your cells. If too much glucose gets into the blood, the extra glucose will be eliminated through your urine. A urine glucose test can be used to help determine if blood glucose levels are too high, which may be a sign of diabetes.

Other names: urine sugar test; urine glucose test; glucosuria test.

What Is It Used For?

A glucose in urine test may be part of a urinalysis, a test that measures different cells, chemicals, and other substances in your urine. Urinalysis is often included as part of a routine exam. A glucose in urine test may also be used to screen for diabetes. However, a urine glucose test is not as accurate as a blood glucose test. It may be ordered if blood glucose testing is difficult or not possible. Some people cannot get blood drawn because their veins are too small or too scarred from repeated punctures. Other people avoid blood tests due to extreme anxiety or fear of needles.

Why Do I Need a Glucose in Urine Test?

You may get a glucose in urine test as part of your regular checkup or if you have symptoms of diabetes and cannot take a blood glucose test. Symptoms of diabetes include:

About This Chapter: This chapter includes text excerpted from "Glucose in Urine Test," MedlinePlus, National Institutes of Health (NIH), April 15, 2019.

- Increased thirst

- More frequent urination

- Blurred vision

- Fatigue

You may also need a urinalysis, which includes a glucose in urine test, if you are pregnant. If high levels of glucose in urine are found, it may indicate gestational diabetes. Gestational diabetes is form of diabetes that happens only during pregnancy. Blood glucose testing can be used to confirm a diagnosis of gestational diabetes. Most pregnant women are tested for gestational diabetes with a blood glucose test, between their 24th and 28th weeks of pregnancy.

What Happens during a Glucose in Urine Test?

If your urine glucose test is part of a urinalysis, you will need to provide a sample of your urine. During your office visit, you will receive a container in which to collect the urine and special instructions to ensure the sample is sterile. These instructions are often referred to as the "clean catch method." The clean catch method includes the following steps:

- Wash your hands.

- Clean your genital area with a cleansing pad. Men should wipe the tip of their penis. Women should open their labia and clean from front to back.

- Start to urinate into the toilet.

- Move the collection container under your urine stream.

- Collect at least an ounce or two of urine into the container, which should have markings to indicate the amount.

- Finish urinating into the toilet.

- Return the sample container as instructed by your healthcare provider.

Your healthcare provider may ask you to monitor your urine glucose at home with a test kit. She or he will provide you with either a kit or a recommendation of which kit to buy. Your urine glucose test kit will include instructions on how to perform the test and a package of strips for testing. Be sure to follow the kit instructions carefully, and talk to your healthcare provider if you have any questions.

Will I Need to Do Anything to Prepare for the Test?

You do not need any special preparations for this test.

Are There Any Risks to the Test?

There is no known risk of having glucose in a urine test.

What Do the Results Mean?

Glucose is not normally found in urine. If results show glucose, it may be a sign of:

- Diabetes

- Pregnancy. As many half of all pregnant women have some glucose in their urine during pregnancy. Too much glucose may indicate gestational diabetes.

- A kidney disorder

- A urine glucose test is only a screening test. If glucose is found in your urine, your provider will order a blood glucose test to help make a diagnosis.

Chapter 17

Ketones in Urine Test

Diabetes is a common chronic condition, and as of 2015, approximately 30 million persons in the United States had diabetes (23 million with diagnosed and 7 million with undiagnosed). Diabetic ketoacidosis (DKA) is a life-threatening but preventable complication of diabetes characterized by uncontrolled hyperglycemia (more than 250 mg/dL), metabolic acidosis, and increased ketone concentration that occurs most frequently in persons with type 1 diabetes. The Centers for Disease Control and Prevention's (CDC) United States Diabetes Surveillance System (USDSS) indicated an increase in hospitalization rates for DKA during 2009–2014, most notably in persons aged younger than 45 years of age.

What Is a Ketones in Urine Test?

The test measures ketone levels in your urine. Normally, your body burns glucose (sugar) for energy. If your cells do not get enough glucose, your body burns fat for energy instead. This produces a substance called "ketones," which can show up in your blood and urine. High ketone levels in urine may indicate diabetic ketoacidosis (DKA), a complication of diabetes that can lead to a coma or even death. A ketones in urine test can prompt you to get treatment before a medical emergency occurs.

About This Chapter: Text in this chapter begins with excerpts from "Trends in Diabetic Ketoacidosis Hospitalizations and In-Hospital Mortality—United States, 2000–2014," Centers for Disease Control and Prevention (CDC), March 29, 2018; Text beginning with the heading "What Is a Ketones in Urine Test?" is excerpted from "Ketones in Urine," MedlinePlus, National Institutes of Health (NIH), April 15, 2019.

What Is It Used For?

The test is often used to help monitor people at a higher risk of developing ketones. These include people with type 1 or type 2 diabetes. If you have diabetes, ketones in urine can mean that you are not getting enough insulin. If you do not have diabetes, you may still be at risk for developing ketones if you:

- Experience chronic vomiting and/or diarrhea

- Have a digestive disorder

- Participate in strenuous exercise

- Are on a very low-carbohydrate diet

- Have an eating disorder

- Are pregnant

Why Do I Need a Ketones in Urine Test?

Your healthcare provider may order a ketones in urine test if you have diabetes or other risk factors for developing ketones. You may also need this test if you have symptoms of ketoacidosis. These include:

- Nausea or vomiting

- Abdominal pain

- Confusion

- Trouble breathing

- Feeling extremely sleepy

People with type 1 diabetes are at a higher risk for ketoacidosis.

What Happens during a Ketones in Urine Test?

A ketones in urine test can be done in the home, as well as in a lab. If in a lab, you will be given instructions to provide a "clean catch" sample. The clean catch method generally includes the following steps:

1. Wash your hands.

2. Clean your genital area with a cleansing pad. Men should wipe the tip of their penis. Women should open their labia, and clean from front to back.

3. Start to urinate into the toilet.

4. Move the collection container under your urine stream.

5. Collect at least an ounce or two of urine into the container, which should have markings to indicate the amount.

6. Finish urinating into the toilet.

7. Return the sample container as instructed by your healthcare provider.

If you do the test at home, follow the instructions that are in your test kit. Your kit will include a package of strips for testing. You will either be instructed to provide a clean catch sample in a container, as described above, or to put the test strip directly in the stream of your urine. Talk to your healthcare provider about specific instructions.

Ketones Test at Home

Purchase urine dip test sticks to test for ketones. Urine testing for ketones is a very important tool especially when your diabetes is out of control or when you are sick. Ketones can be a sign of serious problems that can lead to a diabetic coma.

Ketone test strips can be found at the same places you get other diabetes supplies. They are easy to use.

To use them:

- Dip a ketone test strip into a sample of urine.
- Wait the number of seconds the instructions say. The color of the pad on the strip will change if there are ketones in the urine.
- Compare the color of the pad to the color chart on the bottle or box.
- Record the test result on your testing log.

(Source: "Diabetes Planned Visit Notebook," Agency for Healthcare Research and Quality (AHRQ).)

Will I Need to Do Anything to Prepare for the Test?

You may have to fast (not eat or drink) for a certain period of time before taking a ketones in urine test. Ask your healthcare provider if you need to fast or do any other type of preparation before your test.

Are There Any Risks to the Test?

There is no known risk involved in having a ketones in urine test.

What Do the Results Mean?

Your test results may be a specific number or listed as a "small," "moderate," or "large" amount of ketones. Normal results can vary, depending on your diet, activity level, and other factors. Because high ketone levels can be dangerous, be sure to talk to your healthcare provider about what is normal for you and what your results mean.

Is There Anything Else I Need to Know about a Ketones in Urine Test?

Ketone test kits are available at most pharmacies without a prescription. If you are planning to test for ketones at home, ask your healthcare provider for recommendations on which kit would be best for you. At-home urine tests are easy to perform and can provide accurate results as long as you carefully follow all instructions.

Chapter 18

Diabetes Medicines

Taking insulin or other diabetes medicines is often a part of treating diabetes. Along with healthy food choices and physical activity, medicine can help you manage the disease. Some other treatment options are also available.

What Medicines Might I Take for Diabetes?

The medicine you take will vary by your type of diabetes and how well the medicine controls your blood glucose levels, also called "blood sugar." Other factors, such as your other health conditions, medication costs, and your daily schedule, may play a role in what diabetes medicine you take.

Type 1 Diabetes

If you have type 1 diabetes, you must take insulin because your body no longer makes this hormone. You will need to take insulin several times during the day, including at meals. You also could use an insulin pump, which gives you small, steady doses throughout the day.

Type 2 Diabetes

Some people with type 2 diabetes can manage their disease by making healthy food choices and being more physically active. Many people with type 2 diabetes need diabetes medicines

---

About This Chapter: Text in this chapter begins with excerpts from "Insulin, Medicines, and Other Diabetes Treatments," National Institute of Diabetes and Digestive and Kidney Diseases (NIDDK), November 2016; Text under the heading "U.S. Food and Drug Administration Approves New Treatment for Pediatric Patients with Type 2 Diabetes" is excerpted from "FDA Approves New Treatment for Pediatric Patients with Type 2 Diabetes," U.S. Food and Drug Administration (FDA), June 17, 2019.

as well. These medicines may include diabetes pills or medicines you inject under your skin, such as insulin. In time, you may need more than one diabetes medicine to control your blood glucose. Even if you do not take insulin, you may need it at special times, such as during pregnancy or if you are in the hospital.

Gestational Diabetes

If you have gestational diabetes, you should first try to control your blood glucose level by making healthy food choices and getting regular physical activity. If you cannot reach your blood glucose target, your healthcare team will talk with you about diabetes medicines, such as insulin or the diabetes pill metformin, that may be safe for you to take during pregnancy. Your healthcare team may start you on diabetes medicines right away if your blood glucose is very high.

No matter what type of diabetes you have, taking diabetes medicines every day can feel like a burden sometimes. You may also need medicines for other health problems, such as high blood pressure or high cholesterol, as part of your diabetes care plan.

What Are the Different Types of Insulin?

Several types of insulin are available. Each type starts to work at a different speed, known as "onset," and its effects last a different length of time, known as "duration." Most types of insulin reach a peak, which is when they have the strongest effect. Then, the effects of insulin wear off over the next few hours or so.

Table 18.1. Types of Insulin and How They Work

Insulin Type	How Fast It Starts to Work (Onset)	When It Peaks	How Long It Lasts (Duration)
Rapid-acting	About 15 minutes after injection	1 hour	2 to 4 hours
Short-acting, also called regular	Within 30 minutes after injection	2 to 3 hours	3 to 6 hours
Intermediate-acting	2 to 4 hours after injection	4 to 12 hours	12 to 18 hours
Long-acting	Several hours after injection	Does not peak	24 hours; some last longer

The chart above gives averages. Follow your doctor's advice on when and how to take your insulin. Your doctor might also recommend premixed insulin, which is a mix of two types of insulin. Some types of insulin cost more than others, so talk with your doctor about your options if you are concerned about cost.

What Oral Medicines Treat Type 2 Diabetes?

You may need medicines along with healthy eating and physical activity habits to manage your type 2 diabetes. You can take many diabetes medicines by mouth. These medicines are called "oral medicines."

Most people with type 2 diabetes start medical treatment with metformin pills. Metformin also comes as a liquid. Metformin lowers the amount of glucose that your liver makes and helps your body use insulin better. This drug may help you lose a small amount of weight.

Other oral medicines act in different ways to lower blood glucose levels. You may need to add another diabetes medicine after a while or use a combination treatment. Combining two or three kinds of diabetes medicines can lower blood glucose levels more than taking just one.

What Injectable Medicines Treat Type 2 Diabetes?

Besides insulin, other types of injected medicines are available. These medicines help keep your blood glucose level from going too high after you eat. They may make you feel less hungry and help you lose some weight. Other injectable medicines are not substitutes for insulin.

Other Treatment Options for Diabetes

When medicines and lifestyle changes are not enough to manage your diabetes, a less common treatment may be an option. Other treatments include bariatric surgery for certain people with type 1 or type 2 diabetes, and an "artificial pancreas" and pancreatic islet transplantation for some people with type 1 diabetes.

(Source: "Insulin, Medicines, and Other Diabetes," National Institute of Diabetes and Digestive and Kidney Diseases (NIDDK).)

What Should I Know about Side Effects of Diabetes Medicines?

Side effects are problems that result from medicine. Some diabetes medicines can cause hypoglycemia, also called "low blood glucose," if you do not balance your medicines with food and activity.

Ask your doctor whether your diabetes medicine can cause hypoglycemia or other side effects, such as an upset stomach and weight gain. Take your diabetes medicines as your healthcare professional has instructed you to help prevent side effects and diabetes problems.

U.S. Food and Drug Administration Approves New Treatment for Pediatric Patients with Type 2 Diabetes

The U.S. Food and Drug Administration (FDA) approved Victoza (liraglutide) injection for treatment of pediatric patients 10 years or older with type 2 diabetes. Victoza is the first noninsulin drug approved to treat type 2 diabetes in pediatric patients since metformin was approved for pediatric use in 2000. Victoza has been approved to treat adult patients with type 2 diabetes since 2010.

"The FDA encourages drugs to be made available to the widest number of patients possible when there is evidence of safety and efficacy," said Lisa Yanoff, M.D, acting director of the Division of Metabolism and Endocrinology Products in the FDA's Center for Drug Evaluation and Research. "Victoza has now been shown to improve blood sugar control in pediatric patients with type 2 diabetes. The expanded indication provides an additional treatment option at a time when an increasing number of children are being diagnosed with this disease."

Type 2 diabetes is the most common form of diabetes, occurring when the pancreas cannot make enough insulin to keep blood sugar at normal levels. Although type 2 diabetes primarily occurs in patients over the age of 45, the prevalence rate among younger patients has been rising dramatically over the past couple of decades. The Diabetes Report Card published by the U.S. Centers for Disease Control and Prevention estimates that more than 5,000 new cases of type 2 diabetes are diagnosed each year among U.S. youth younger than age 20.

Victoza improves blood sugar levels by creating the same effects in the body as the glucagon-like peptide (GLP-1) receptor protein in the pancreas. GLP-1 is often found in insufficient levels in type 2 diabetes patients. Like GLP-1, Victoza slows digestion, prevents the liver from making too much glucose (a simple sugar), and helps the pancreas produce more insulin when needed. As noted on the label, Victoza is not a substitute for insulin and is not indicated for patients with type 1 diabetes or those with diabetic ketoacidosis, a condition associated with diabetes where the body breaks down fat too quickly because there is inadequate insulin or none at all. Victoza is also indicated to reduce the risk of major adverse cardiovascular events in adults with type 2 diabetes and established cardiovascular disease; however, its effect on major adverse cardiovascular events in pediatrics was not studied and it is not indicated for this use in children.

The efficacy and safety of Victoza for reducing blood sugar in patients with type 2 diabetes was studied in several placebo-controlled trials in adults and one placebo-controlled trial with 134 pediatric patients 10 years and older for more than 26 weeks. Approximately 64 percent of patients in the pediatric study had a reduction in their hemoglobin A1c (HbA1c) below 7 percent while on Victoza, compared to only 37 percent who achieved these results with the placebo. HbA1c is a blood test that is routinely performed to evaluate how well a patient's diabetes is controlled, and a lower number indicates better control of the disease. These results occurred regardless of whether the patient also took insulin at the same time. Adult patients who took Victoza with insulin or other drugs that increase the amount of insulin the body makes (e.g., sulfonylurea) may have an increased risk of hypoglycemia (low blood sugar). Meanwhile, pediatric patients 10 years and older taking Victoza had a higher risk of hypoglycemia regardless of whether they took other therapies for diabetes.

The prescribing information for Victoza includes a Boxed Warning to advise healthcare professionals and patients about the increased risk of thyroid C-cell tumors. For this reason, patients who have had, or have family members who have ever had medullary thyroid carcinoma (MTC) should not use Victoza, nor should patients who have an endocrine system condition called "multiple endocrine neoplasia syndrome type 2" (MEN 2). In addition, people who have a prior serious hypersensitivity reaction to Victoza or any of the product components should not use Victoza. Victoza also carries warnings about pancreatitis, Victoza pen sharing, hypoglycemia when used in conjunction with certain other drugs known to cause hypoglycemia including insulin and sulfonylurea, renal impairment or kidney failure, hypersensitivity and acute gallbladder disease. The most common side effects are nausea, diarrhea, vomiting, decreased appetite, indigestion and constipation.

The FDA granted this application Priority Review. The approval of Victoza was granted to Novo Nordisk.

The FDA, an agency within the U.S. Department of Health and Human Services, protects the public health by assuring the safety, effectiveness, and security of human and veterinary drugs, vaccines and other biological products for human use, and medical devices. The agency also is responsible for the safety and security of our nation's food supply, cosmetics, dietary supplements, products that give off electronic radiation, and for regulating tobacco products.

Chapter 19

Insulin Delivery Devices

Insulin: An Overview[1]

Insulin helps to take the sugar in your blood to other parts of your body. Diabetes affects how your body makes or uses insulin. Diabetes can make it hard to control how much sugar is in your blood.

Available Devices for Taking Insulin[2]

Many people with diabetes must take insulin to manage their disease. Most people who take insulin use a needle and syringe to inject insulin just under the skin. Several other devices for taking insulin are available, and new approaches are under development. No matter which approach a person uses for taking insulin, consistent monitoring of blood glucose levels is important. Alternative devices for taking insulin are as follows.

Insulin pens provide a convenient, easy-to-use way of injecting insulin and may be less painful than a standard needle and syringe. An insulin pen looks like a pen with a cartridge. Some of these devices use replaceable cartridges of insulin. Other pens are prefilled with insulin and are totally disposable after the insulin is injected. Insulin pen users screw a short, fine, disposable needle on the tip of the pen before an injection. Then, users turn a dial to select the desired dose of insulin, inject the needle, and press a plunger on the end to deliver the insulin just under the skin. Insulin pens are less widely used in the United States than in many other countries.

About This Chapter: This chapter includes text excerpted from documents published by two public domain sources. Text under the headings marked 1 are excerpted from "Insulin," U.S. Food and Drug Administration (FDA), May 22, 2019; Text under the headings marked 2 are excerpted from "Alternative Devices for Taking Insulin," National Institute of Diabetes and Digestive and Kidney Diseases (NIDDK), May 2009. Reviewed June 2019.

External insulin pumps are typically about the size of a deck of cards or cell phones, weigh about 3 ounces, and can be worn on a belt or carried in a pocket. Most pumps use a disposable plastic cartridge as an insulin reservoir. A needle and plunger are temporarily attached to the cartridge to allow the user to fill the cartridge with insulin from a vial. The user then removes the needle and plunger, and loads the filled cartridge into the pump. Disposable infusion sets are used with insulin pumps to deliver insulin to an infusion site on the body, such as the abdomen. Infusion sets include a cannula—a needle or a small, soft tube—that the user inserts into the tissue beneath the skin. Devices are available to help insert the cannula. Narrow, flexible plastic tubing carries insulin from the pump to the infusion site. On the skin's surface, an adhesive patch or dressing holds the infusion set in place until the user replaces it after a few days.

Users set the pumps to give a steady trickle or "basal" amount of insulin continuously throughout the day. Pumps can also give "bolus" doses—one-time larger doses—of insulin at meals and at times when blood glucose is too high based on the programming set by the user. Frequent blood glucose monitoring is essential to determine insulin dosages and to ensure that insulin is delivered.

Injection ports provide an alternative to daily injections. Injection ports look like infusion sets without the long tubing. As with infusion sets, injection ports have a cannula that is inserted into the tissue beneath the skin. On the skin's surface, an adhesive patch or dressing holds the port in place. The user injects insulin through the port with a needle and syringe or an insulin pen. The port remains in place for several days and is then replaced. The use of an injection port allows a person to reduce the number of skin punctures to one every few days to apply a new port.

Action Steps—If You Take Insulin

Keep a daily record of:

- Your blood glucose levels
- The times of day you take insulin
- The amount and type of insulin you take
- What types of physical activity you do and for how long
- When and what you eat
- Whether you have ketones in your blood or urine
- When you are sick

(Source: "Monitor Your Diabetes," National Institute of Diabetes and Digestive and Kidney Diseases (NIDDK).)

Injection aids are devices that help users give injections with needles and syringes through the use of spring-loaded syringe holders or stabilizing guides. Many injection aids have a button the user pushes to inject the insulin.

Insulin jet injectors send a fine spray of insulin into the skin at high pressure instead of using a needle to deliver the insulin.

Insulin Safety Tips[1]

- Never drink insulin.

- Do not share insulin needles, pens, or cartridges with anyone else.

- Talk to your doctor before you change or stop using your insulin.

- Do not inject your insulin in the exact same spot each time.

- Throw away needles in a hard container that can be closed like a laundry detergent bottle.

- Check the expiration date on the insulin before you use it.

- Plan how to take care of your insulin when you travel and during an emergency.

What Are the Prospects for an Artificial Pancreas?[2]

To overcome the limitations of current insulin therapy, researchers have long sought to link glucose monitoring and insulin delivery by developing an artificial pancreas. An artificial pancreas is a system that will mimic, as closely as possible, the way a healthy pancreas detects changes in blood glucose levels and responds automatically to secrete appropriate amounts of insulin. Although not a cure, an artificial pancreas has the potential to significantly improve diabetes care and management, and to reduce the burden of monitoring and managing blood glucose.

An artificial pancreas based on mechanical devices requires at least three components:

- A continuous glucose monitoring (CGM) system

- An insulin delivery system

- A computer program that adjusts insulin delivery based on changes in glucose levels

Continuous glucose monitoring systems approved by the U.S. Food and Drug Administration (FDA) include those made by Abbott, DexCom, and Medtronic. A CGM system paired with an insulin pump is available from Medtronic. This integrated system, called the "Minimed Paradigm REAL-Time System," is not an artificial pancreas, but it does represent the first step in joining glucose monitoring and insulin delivery systems using the most advanced technology available.

Points to Remember

- Many people with diabetes who need insulin use a needle and syringe to inject insulin under the skin.

- The most common alternative ways to deliver insulin are insulin pens and insulin pumps. Injection ports, injection aids, and insulin jet injectors are also available.

- Researchers are developing an artificial pancreas, a system of mechanical devices that will automatically adjust insulin delivery based on changes in glucose levels.

- People who take insulin should monitor their blood glucose levels regularly.

- Good glucose control can prevent complications of diabetes.

Chapter 20

Managing Hypoglycemia

What Is Hypoglycemia?

Hypoglycemia, also called "low blood glucose" or "low blood sugar," occurs when the level of glucose in your blood drops below normal. For many people with diabetes, that means a level of 70 milligrams per deciliter (mg/dL) or less. Your numbers might be different, so check with your healthcare provider to find out what level is too low for you.

There are two ways to measure blood sugar.

- Blood sugar checks that you do yourself. These tell you what your blood sugar level is at the time you test. You use a blood glucose meter to check your blood sugar. This device uses a small drop of blood from your finger to measure your blood sugar level. You can get the meter and supplies in a drug store or by mail.

- The A1C (A-one-C) is a test done in a lab or at your provider's office. This test tells you your average blood sugar level over the past 2 to 3 months.

(Source: "Know Your Blood Sugar Numbers: Use Them to Manage Your Diabetes," National Institute of Diabetes and Digestive and Kidney Diseases (NIDDK).)

What Are the Symptoms of Hypoglycemia?

Symptoms of hypoglycemia tend to come on quickly and can vary from person to person. You may have one or more mild-to-moderate symptoms as listed below. Sometimes, people do not feel any symptoms.

About This Chapter: This chapter includes text excerpted from "Low Blood Glucose (Hypoglycemia)," National Institute of Diabetes and Digestive and Kidney Diseases (NIDDK), August 2016.

Severe hypoglycemia is when your blood glucose level becomes so low that you are unable to treat yourself and need help from another person. Severe hypoglycemia is dangerous and needs to be treated right away. This condition is more common in people with type 1 diabetes.

Mild-to-Moderate Hypoglycemia

- Shaky or jittery
- Sweaty
- Hungry
- Headache
- Blurred vision
- Sleepy or tired
- Dizzy or light-headed
- Confused or disoriented
- Pale
- Uncoordinated
- Irritable or nervous
- Argumentative or combative
- Changed behavior or personality
- Trouble concentrating
- Weak
- Fast or irregular heartbeat

Severe Hypoglycemia

- Unable to eat or drink
- Seizures or convulsions (jerky movements)
- Unconsciousness

Some symptoms of hypoglycemia during sleep are:

- Crying out or having nightmares

- Sweating enough to make your pajamas or sheets damp

- Feeling tired, irritable, or confused after waking up

What Causes Hypoglycemia in Diabetes

Hypoglycemia can be a side effect of insulin or other types of diabetes medicines that help your body make more insulin. Two types of diabetes pills can cause hypoglycemia: sulfonylureas and meglitinides. Ask your healthcare team if your diabetes medicine can cause hypoglycemia.

Although other diabetes medicines do not cause hypoglycemia by themselves, they can increase the chances of hypoglycemia if you also take insulin, a sulfonylurea, or a meglitinide.

What Other Factors Contribute to Hypoglycemia In Diabetes?

If you take insulin or diabetes medicines that increase the amount of insulin your body makes but do not match your medications with your food or physical activity, you could develop hypoglycemia. The following factors can make hypoglycemia more likely.

Not Eating Enough Carbohydrates

When you eat foods containing carbohydrates (carbs), your digestive system breaks down the sugars and starches into glucose. Glucose then enters your bloodstream and raises your blood glucose level. If you do not eat enough carbohydrates to match your medication, your blood glucose could drop too low.

Skipping or Delaying a Meal

If you skip or delay a meal, your blood glucose could drop too low. Hypoglycemia also can occur when you are asleep and have not eaten for several hours.

Increasing Physical Activity

Increasing your physical activity level beyond your normal routine can lower your blood glucose level for up to 24 hours after the activity.

Drinking Too Much Alcohol without Enough Food

Alcohol makes it harder for your body to keep your blood glucose level steady, especially if you have not eaten in a while. The effects of alcohol can also keep you from feeling the symptoms of hypoglycemia, which may lead to severe hypoglycemia.

Being Sick

When you are sick, you may not be able to eat as much or keep food down, which can cause low blood glucose.

How Can I Prevent Hypoglycemia If I Have Diabetes?

If you are taking insulin, a sulfonylurea, or a meglitinide, using your diabetes management plan and working with your healthcare team to adjust your plan as needed can help you prevent hypoglycemia. The following actions can also help prevent hypoglycemia:

Check Blood Glucose Levels

Knowing your blood glucose level can help you decide how much medicine to take, what food to eat, and how physically active to be. To find out your blood glucose level, check yourself with a blood glucose meter as often as your doctor advises.

Sometimes, people with diabetes do not feel or recognize the symptoms of hypoglycemia, a problem called "hypoglycemia unawareness." If you have had hypoglycemia without feeling any symptoms, you may need to check your blood glucose more often so you know when you need to treat your hypoglycemia or take steps to prevent it. Be sure to check your blood glucose before you drive.

If you have hypoglycemia unawareness or have hypoglycemia often, ask your healthcare provider about a continuous glucose monitor (CGM). A CGM checks your blood glucose level at regular times throughout the day and night. CGMs can tell you if your blood glucose is falling quickly and sound an alarm if your blood glucose falls too low. CGM alarms can wake you up if you have hypoglycemia during sleep.

Eat Regular Meals and Snacks

Your meal plan is key to preventing hypoglycemia. Eat regular meals and snacks with the correct amount of carbohydrates to help keep your blood glucose level from going too low. Also, if you drink alcoholic beverages, it is best to eat some food at the same time.

Be Physically Active Safely

Physical activity can lower your blood glucose during the activity and for hours afterward. To help prevent hypoglycemia, you may need to check your blood glucose before, during, and after physical activity, and adjust your medicine or carbohydrate intake. For example, you might eat a snack before being physically active or decrease your insulin dose as directed by your healthcare provider to keep your blood glucose from dropping too low.

Work with Your Healthcare Team

Tell your healthcare team if you have had hypoglycemia. Your healthcare team may adjust your diabetes medicines or other aspects of your management plan. Learn about balancing your medicines, eating plan, and physical activity to prevent hypoglycemia. Ask if you should have a glucagon emergency kit to carry with you at all times.

How Do I Treat Hypoglycemia?

If you begin to feel 1 or more hypoglycemia symptoms, check your blood glucose. If your blood glucose level is below your target or less than 70, eat or drink 15 grams of carbohydrates right away. Examples include:

- 4 glucose tablets or 1 tube of glucose gel
- ½ cup (4 ounces) of fruit juice—not low-calorie or reduced sugar*
- ½ can (4 to 6 ounces) of soda—not low-calorie or reduced sugar
- 1 tablespoon of sugar, honey, or corn syrup
- 2 tablespoons of raisins

Wait 15 minutes and check your blood glucose again. If your glucose level is still low, eat or drink another 15 grams of glucose or carbohydrates. Check your blood glucose again after another 15 minutes. Repeat these steps until your glucose level is back to normal.

If your next meal is more than one hour away, have a snack to keep your blood glucose level in your target range. Try crackers or a piece of fruit.

People who have kidney disease should not drink orange juice for their 15 grams of carbohydrates because it contains a lot of potassium. Apple, grape, or cranberry juice are good options.

Treating Hypoglycemia If You Take Acarbose or Miglitol

If you take acarbose or miglitol along with diabetes medicines that can cause hypoglycemia, you will need to take glucose tablets or glucose gel if your blood glucose level is too low. Eating or drinking other sources of carbohydrates will not raise your blood glucose level quickly enough.

What If I Have Severe Hypoglycemia and Cannot Treat Myself?

Someone will need to give you a glucagon injection if you have severe hypoglycemia. An injection of glucagon will quickly raise your blood glucose level. Talk with your healthcare provider about when and how to use a glucagon emergency kit. If you have an emergency kit, check the date on the package to make sure it has not expired.

If you are likely to have severe hypoglycemia, teach your family, friends, and coworkers when and how to give you a glucagon injection. Also, tell your family, friends, and coworkers to call 911 right away after giving you a glucagon injection or if you do not have a glucagon emergency kit with you.

If you have hypoglycemia often or have had severe hypoglycemia, you should wear a medical alert bracelet or pendant. A medical alert ID tells other people that you have diabetes and need care right away. Getting prompt care can help prevent the serious problems that hypoglycemia can cause.

Chapter 21

Managing Hyperglycemia

Recognizing Hyperglycemia

Hyperglycemia means blood glucose levels are above the target range, as specified in the student's Diabetes Medical Management Plan (DMMP), as created by the American Diabetes Association (ADA). Almost all patients with diabetes will experience blood glucose levels above their target range at times throughout the day. For many students, these elevations in blood glucose will be only minimally above the target range (less than 250 mg/dL) and are short in duration. Other students may experience daily spikes of blood glucose levels that are high (in excess of 250 mg/dL) and of longer duration.

Hyperglycemia does not usually result in a medical emergency. Hyperglycemia may be caused by too little insulin or other blood glucose-lowering medications, a malfunction in the insulin pump or infusion set, food intake that has not been covered adequately by insulin or other blood glucose-lowering medications, or decreased physical activity. Other causes include illness, infection, injury, or severe physical or emotional stress. Onset of hyperglycemia may occur over several hours or days.

Hyperglycemia Symptoms

Symptoms of hyperglycemia include increased thirst, dry mouth, frequent or increased urination, change in appetite, blurry vision, and fatigue. In the short term, hyperglycemia can impair cognitive abilities and adversely affect academic performance. In the long term,

---

About This Chapter: This chapter includes text excerpted from "How to Help Students Implement Effective Diabetes Management," National Institute of Diabetes and Digestive and Kidney Diseases (NIDDK), December 19, 2015. Reviewed June 2019.

moderately high blood glucose levels can increase the risk for serious complications, such as heart disease, stroke, blindness, kidney failure, nerve disease, gum disease, and amputations.

Hyperglycemia Treatment

Treatment of hyperglycemia begins with checking the patient's blood glucose level to determine if it is above the target range. When checking blood glucose at a time not specified in the DMMP, treatment decisions should take into account the time and amount of the student's last carbohydrate intake or insulin dose.

In accordance with the Emergency Care Plan for Hyperglycemia, a two-page form also from the ADA—the patient's urine or blood should be checked for ketones, the chemicals the body makes when there is not enough insulin in the blood and the body must break down fat for energy. The urine ketone test involves dipping a special strip into the urine, waiting for a specified amount of time, and then comparing the resulting color to a color chart. The blood ketone test is done with a finger stick using a special meter and a test strip, similar to checking blood glucose. Patients with type 2 diabetes usually still make a reasonable amount of insulin, and therefore, ketone checks may not be prescribed.

Ketones and Diabetic Ketoacidosis

While hyperglycemia does not usually result in a medical emergency, the following situations may lead to a breakdown of fat, causing ketones to form along with the hyperglycemia:

- Significant or prolonged insulin deficiency from failure to take any insulin or the correct amount of insulin

- An insulin pump or infusion set malfunction causing an interruption in insulin delivery

- Physical or emotional stress that increases the release of hormones that work against the action of insulin

- Infection or illness, particularly with diarrhea and/or vomiting

Ketones are usually associated with high blood glucose levels but also may occur when a student is ill and blood glucose levels fall below the student's target range. At first, ketones will be cleared by the kidneys into the urine, but as their production increases, they build up in the bloodstream causing diabetic ketoacidosis (DKA), a medical emergency.

Diabetic ketoacidosis develops over hours to days and is associated with hyperglycemia and dehydration. As a result of these conditions, the classic signs of diabetic ketoacidosis include severe abdominal pain; nausea and vomiting; fruity breath, heavy breathing, or shortness of breath; chest pain; increasing sleepiness or lethargy; and depressed level of consciousness.

Checklist for the Treatment of Hyperglycemia for Teachers and School Professionals

- Refer to the student's DMMP for specific instructions.
- Check the blood glucose level to determine if it is high.
- Check urine or blood for ketones.
- Calculate the insulin correction dose needed.
- Administer supplemental insulin dose in accordance with the student's Emergency Care Plan for Hyperglycemia. (If a student uses an insulin pump, see instructions below.)
- Give extra water or nonsugar-containing drinks (as needed).
- Allow free and unrestricted access to the restroom and to liquids, as high blood glucose levels can cause increased urination and may lead to dehydration if the student cannot replace the fluids.
- Recheck blood glucose every 2 hours to determine if it is decreasing to target range.
- Restrict participation in physical activity as specified in the DMMP. However, if the student is not nauseous or vomiting and moderate to large ketones are not present, light physical activity might help to lower the blood glucose level.
- Notify parents/guardians as specified in the DMMP.

Checklist for Students Using an Insulin Pump

- If a student uses a pump, check to see if the pump is connected properly and functioning by giving a correction bolus through the pump and checking blood glucose level 1 hour later.
- If moderate or large ketones are present, change pump site and treat ketones with an injection of insulin by syringe or insulin pen.
- For infusion site failure: Insert new infusion set and/or replace reservoir, or give insulin by syringe or insulin pen.
- For suspected pump failure: Suspend or remove the pump and give insulin by syringe or insulin pen.

Chapter 22

Beware of Diabetes Treatment Fraud

Beware of Illegally Marketed Diabetes Treatments

As the number of people diagnosed with diabetes continues to grow, illegally marketed products promising to prevent, treat, and even cure diabetes are flooding the marketplace.

The U.S. Food and Drug Administration (FDA) is advising consumers not to use such products—for many reasons. For example, they may contain harmful ingredients or may improperly be marketed as over-the-counter (OTC) products when they should be marketed as prescription products. Illegally marketed products carry an additional risk if they cause people to delay or discontinue effective treatments for diabetes. Without proper disease management, people with diabetes are at a greater risk for developing serious health complications.

More than 30 million people in the United States have diabetes, and one out of four do not know they have it, according to the Centers for Disease Control and Prevention (CDC). Millions more have prediabetes, meaning they have higher than normal blood sugar levels and can reduce their risks of developing diabetes through healthy lifestyle changes, including diet and exercise.

"People with chronic or incurable diseases may feel desperate and become easy targets. Bogus products for diabetes are particularly troubling because there are effective options available to help manage this serious disease rather than exposing patients to unproven and

About This Chapter: This chapter includes text excerpted from "Beware of Illegally Marketed Diabetes Treatments," U.S. Food and Drug Administration (FDA), May 11, 2017.

unreasonably risky products," said Jason Humbert, a captain with the U.S. Public Health Service (USPHS) who is with the FDA's Office of Regulatory Affairs (ORA). "Failure to follow well-established treatment plans can lead to, among other things, amputations, kidney disease, blindness, and death."

To protect the public health, the FDA surveys the marketplace for illegally marketed products promising to treat diabetes and its complications, and investigates consumer complaints.

Health fraud involves selling drugs, devices, foods, or cosmetics that have not been proven effective. Keep in mind—if it sounds too good to be true, it's probably a scam. At best, these scams don't work. At worst, they're dangerous. They also waste money, and they might keep you from getting the treatment you really need.

To protect yourself, recognize the red flags such as:

- Miracle cure
- Quick fix
- Ancient remedy
- Secret ingredient
- Scientific breakthrough

Before taking an unproven or little known treatment, talk to a doctor or healthcare professional—especially when taking prescription drugs.

(Source: "Health Fraud," MedlinePlus, National Institutes of Health (NIH).)

Unapproved Diabetes Drugs

The FDA has issued warning letters to various companies that market products for diabetes in violation of federal law. These products were marketed as dietary supplements; alternative medicines, such as ayurvedics; prescription drugs; OTC drugs; and homeopathic products. Some of the companies also promoted the same unapproved drugs for other serious diseases, including cancer, sexually transmitted diseases, and macular degeneration.

FDA laboratory analysis has found "all-natural" products for diabetes to contain undeclared active ingredients found in approved prescription drugs intended for treatment of diabetes. Undeclared active ingredients can cause serious harm. If consumers and their healthcare professionals are unaware of the actual active ingredients in the products they are taking, these products may interact in dangerous ways with other medications. One possible complication: Patients may end up taking a larger combined dose of the diabetic drugs than they intended.

This may cause a significant and unsafe drop in blood sugar levels, a condition known as "hypoglycemia."

The FDA also looks at illegal marketing of prescription drugs by fraudulent online pharmacies. Signs that may indicate an online pharmacy is legitimate include: requiring that patients have a valid prescription, providing a physical address in the United States, being licensed by a state pharmacy board, and providing a state-licensed pharmacist to answer questions.

Some fraudulent online pharmacies illegally market drugs that are not approved in the United States, or sell otherwise approved prescription drug products without meeting necessary requirements. Although some of these websites may offer for sale what appear to be FDA-approved prescription drugs, the FDA cannot be certain that the manufacture or the handling of these drugs follows U.S. regulations or that the drugs are safe and effective for their intended uses. Also, there is a risk the drugs may be counterfeit, contaminated, expired, or otherwise unsafe.

A Far-Reaching Problem

"Products that promise an easy fix might be alluring, but consumers are gambling with their health. In general, diabetes is a chronic disease, but it is manageable. And people can lower their risk for developing complications by following treatments prescribed by healthcare professionals, carefully monitoring blood sugar levels, and sticking to an appropriate diet and exercise program," Humbert said.

Part Three
The Physical Complications of Diabetes

Chapter 23

Diabetes-Related Health Concerns

Diabetes can affect any part of your body. The good news is that you can prevent most of these problems by keeping your blood glucose (blood sugar) under control, eating healthy, being physically active, working with your healthcare provider to keep your blood pressure and cholesterol under control, and getting necessary screening tests.

Heart Disease
How Can Diabetes Affect My Heart?

Heart disease is the leading cause of early death among people with diabetes. Adults with diabetes are 2 to 3 times more likely than people without diabetes to die of heart disease or have a stroke. Also, about 74 percent of people with diabetes have high blood pressure, a risk factor for heart disease.

How Can I Be "Heart Healthy" and Avoid Heart Disease If I Have Diabetes?

To protect your heart and blood vessels:

- Eat healthy—choose a healthy diet, low in salt. Work with a dietitian to plan healthy meals.

About This Chapter: This chapter includes text excerpted from "Prevent Complications," Centers for Disease Control and Prevention (CDC), March 20, 2019.

- Get physically active—if you are overweight, talk to your doctor about how to safely lose weight. Ask about a physical activity or exercise program that would be best for you.

- Do not smoke—quit smoking, if you currently do.

- Maintain healthy blood glucose, blood pressure, and cholesterol levels—get an A1C test at least twice a year to determine what your average blood glucose level was for the past three months. Get your blood pressure checked at every doctor's visit, and get your cholesterol checked at least once a year. Take medications if prescribed by your doctor.

How Are Cholesterol, Triglyceride, Weight, and Blood Pressure Problems Related to Diabetes?

People with type 2 diabetes have high cholesterol and triglyceride rates, obesity, and high blood pressure, all of which are major contributors to higher rates of heart disease. Many people with diabetes have several of these conditions at the same time. This combination is often called "metabolic syndrome." The metabolic syndrome is often defined as the presence of any three of the following conditions:

- Excess weight around the waist

- High levels of triglycerides

- Low levels of high-density lipoprotein (HDL), or "good," cholesterol

- High blood pressure

- High fasting blood glucose levels.

If you have one or more of these conditions, you are at an increased risk for having one or more of the others. The more conditions that you have, the greater the risk to your health.

Kidney Disease
How Can Diabetes Affect the Kidneys?

In diabetic kidney disease (also called "diabetic nephropathy"), cells and blood vessels in the kidneys are damaged, affecting the organs' ability to filter out waste. Waste builds up in your blood instead of being excreted. In some cases, this can lead to kidney failure. When your kidneys fail, you will have to have your blood filtered through a machine (dialysis) several times a week, or you will need a kidney transplant.

How Can I Keep My Kidneys Healthy If I Have Diabetes?

You can do a lot to prevent kidney problems. Controlling your blood glucose and keeping your blood pressure under control can prevent or delay the onset of kidney disease.

Diabetic kidney disease happens slowly and silently, so you might not feel that anything is wrong until severe problems develop. Therefore, it is important to get your blood and urine checked for kidney problems each year.

Your doctor will see how well your kidneys are working by testing every year for microalbumin (a protein) in the urine. Microalbumin in the urine is an early sign of diabetic kidney disease. Your doctor can also do a yearly blood test to measure your kidney function.

If you develop a bladder or kidney infection, visit your doctor. Symptoms include cloudy or bloody urine, pain or burning when you urinate, an urgent need to urinate often, back pain, chills, or fever.

Nerve Damage
How Can Diabetes Affect Nerve Endings?

Having high blood glucose for many years can damage blood vessels that bring oxygen to some nerve endings. Damaged nerves may stop, slow, or send messages at wrong times. Numbness, pain, and weakness in the hands, arms, feet, and legs may develop. Problems may also occur in various organs, including the digestive tract, heart, and sex organs. "Diabetic neuropathy" is the medical term for damage to the nervous system from diabetes. The most common type is peripheral neuropathy, which affects the arms and legs.

An estimated 50 percent of people with diabetes have some nerve problems, but not all have symptoms. Nerve problems can develop at any time, but the longer a person has diabetes, the greater the risk. The highest rates of nerve problems are among people who have had the disease for at least 25 years.

Diabetic nerve problems also are more common in people who have problems controlling their blood glucose levels, blood pressure, weight, and in people over the age of 40.

How Can I Prevent Nerve Damage If I Have Diabetes?

You can help keep your nervous system healthy by keeping your blood glucose as close to normal as possible, getting regular physical activity, not smoking, taking good care of your feet each day, having your healthcare provider examine your feet at least four times a year, and getting your feet tested for nerve damage at least once a year.

Digestive Problems
How Can Diabetes Affect the Digestion?

Gastroparesis (delayed gastric emptying) is a disorder where the stomach takes too long to empty itself due to nerve damage. It frequently occurs in people with either type 1 or type 2 diabetes.

Symptoms of gastroparesis include heartburn, nausea, vomiting of undigested food, an early feeling of fullness when eating, weight loss, abdominal bloating, erratic blood glucose levels, lack of appetite, gastroesophageal reflux, and spasms of the stomach wall.

Foot Problems
Why Is It Especially Important to Take Care of My Feet If I Have Diabetes?

Sometimes nerve damage can deform or misshapen your feet, causing pressure points that can turn into blisters, sores, or ulcers. Poor circulation can make these injuries slow to heal. Sometimes this can lead to amputation of a toe, foot, or leg.

What should I do on a regular basis to take care of my feet?

- Look for cuts, cracks, sores, red spots, swelling, infected toenails, splinters, blisters, and calluses on the feet each day. Call your doctor if such wounds do not heal after one day.

- If you have corns and calluses, ask your doctor or podiatrist about the best way to care for them.

- Wash your feet in warm—not hot—water, and dry them well.

- Cut your toenails once a week or when needed. Cut toenails when they are soft from washing. Cut them to the shape of the toe and not too short. File the edges with an emery board.

- Rub lotion on the tops and bottoms of feet—but not between the toes—to prevent cracking and drying.

- Wear stockings or socks to avoid blisters and sores.

- Wear clean, lightly padded socks that fit well. Seamless socks are best.

- Wear shoes that fit well. Break in new shoes slowly, by wearing them 1 to 2 hours each day for a week to two weeks.

- Always wear shoes or slippers, because when you are barefoot it is easy to step on something and hurt your feet.

- Protect your feet from extreme heat and cold.

- When sitting, keep the blood flowing to your lower limbs by propping your feet up and moving your toes and ankles for a few minutes at a time.

- Avoid smoking, which reduces blood flow to the feet.

- Keep your blood sugar, blood pressure, and cholesterol under control by eating healthy foods, staying active, and taking your diabetes medicines.

Sexual Response and Urinary Tract Infections
How Can Diabetes Affect My Sexual Response?

Many people with diabetic nerve damage have trouble having sex. For example, men can have trouble maintaining an erection and ejaculating. Women can have trouble with sexual response and vaginal lubrication. Both men and women with diabetes can get urinary tract infections (UTIs) and bladder problems more often than average.

Oral Health
How Can Diabetes Affect My Mouth, Teeth, and Gums?

People with diabetes are more likely to have problems with their teeth and gums due to high blood glucose. And like all infections, dental infections can make your blood glucose go up. Sore, swollen, and red gums that bleed when you brush your teeth are a sign of a dental problem called "gingivitis." Another problem, called "periodontitis," happens when your gums shrink or pull away from your teeth.

People with diabetes can have tooth and gum problems more often if their blood glucose stays high. Smoking also makes it more likely for you to have gum disease, especially if you have diabetes and are 45 years of age or older.

How Can I Keep My Mouth, Gums, and Teeth Healthy If I Have Diabetes?

You can help maintain your oral health by:

- Keeping your blood glucose as close to normal as possible

- Brushing your teeth at least twice a day, and flossing once a day

- Keeping any dentures clean

- Getting a dental cleaning and exam twice a year, and telling your dentist that you have diabetes

Call your dentist with any problems, such as gums that are red, sore, bleeding, or pulling away from the teeth; any possible tooth infection; or soreness from dentures.

Vision
How Can Diabetes Affect the Eyes?

In diabetic eye disease, high blood glucose, and high blood pressure cause small blood vessels to swell and leak liquid into the retina of the eye, blurring the vision and sometimes leading to blindness. People with diabetes are also more likely to develop cataracts (a clouding of the eye's lens) and glaucoma (optic nerve damage). Laser surgery can in some cases help these conditions.

How Can I Keep My Eyes Healthy If I Have Diabetes?

There is a lot you can do to prevent eye problems. Keeping your blood glucose level closer to normal can prevent or delay the onset of diabetic eye disease. Also, keeping your blood pressure under control is important. Finding and treating eye problems early can help save your sight.

Have an eye doctor give you a dilated eye exam at least once a year. The doctor will use eye drops to enlarge (dilate) your pupils to examine the backs of your eyes. Your eyes will be checked for signs of cataracts or glaucoma, problems that people with diabetes are more likely to get.

Because diabetic eye disease may develop without symptoms, regular eye exams are important for finding problems early. Some people may notice signs of vision changes. If you are having trouble reading, if your vision is blurred, or if you are seeing rings around lights, dark spots, or flashing lights, you may have eye problems. Be sure to tell your healthcare team or eye doctor about any eye problems you may have.

Mental Health
How Are Diabetes and Mental Health Related?

Untreated mental-health issues can make diabetes harder to handle, and the opposite is also true—getting help for a mental-health problem can help you manage diabetes. But, many do not get the help they need. Problems like depression are much more common in people with diabetes, but only 25 to 50 percent get diagnosed and treated.

Stress is a part of life, but if you are feeling stressed you may not take as good care of yourself as usual. Another very common problem is diabetes distress—feeling discouraged, frustrated, or tired of dealing with diabetes every day. That may lead you to slip into unhealthy habits.

In Charge, But Not Alone

Everyone's diabetes is different. Some people will still have complications even with good control. Maybe that's you—you've been trying hard but not seeing results. Or you've developed a health problem related to diabetes in spite of your best efforts.

You are in the driver's seat when it comes to managing your diabetes—watching what you eat, making time for physical activity, taking meds, checking your blood sugar. Also, be sure to stay in touch with your healthcare team to keep going in the right direction.

If you feel discouraged and frustrated, you may slip into unhealthy habits, stop monitoring your blood sugar, even skip doctors' appointments. That's when your team can help you get back on track, from setting goals and reminding you of your progress to offering new ideas and strategies.

(Source: "Putting the Brakes on Diabetes Complications," Centers for Disease Control and Prevention (CDC).)

Chapter 24

Diabetes, Heart Disease, and Stroke

Having diabetes means that you are more likely to develop heart disease and have a greater chance of a heart attack or a stroke. People with diabetes are also more likely to have certain conditions, or risk factors, that increase the chances of having heart disease or stroke, such as high blood pressure or high cholesterol. If you have diabetes, you can protect your heart and health by managing your blood glucose, also called "blood sugar," as well as your blood pressure and cholesterol. If you smoke, get help to stop.

What Is the Link among Diabetes, Heart Disease, and Stroke?

Over time, high blood glucose from diabetes can damage your blood vessels and the nerves that control your heart and blood vessels. The longer you have diabetes, the higher the chances that you will develop heart disease.

People with diabetes tend to develop heart disease at a younger age than people without diabetes. In adults with diabetes, the most common causes of death are heart disease and stroke. Adults with diabetes are nearly twice as likely to die from heart disease or stroke as people without diabetes.

The good news is that the steps you take to manage your diabetes also help to lower your chances of having heart disease or stroke.

About This Chapter: This chapter includes text excerpted from "Diabetes, Heart Disease, and Stroke," National Institute of Diabetes and Digestive and Kidney Diseases (NIDDK), February 2017.

> ### Diabetes, Heart Disease, Stroke, and Women
>
> Women with diabetes have a 40 percent greater risk of developing heart disease and a 25 percent greater risk of stroke than men with diabetes do. Experts are not sure why the risk is so much greater in women with diabetes than in men with diabetes. Women's biology may play a role: Women usually have more body fat, which can put them at greater risk for heart disease and stroke. If you are a woman with diabetes, you can take steps to control your condition and improve your chances of avoiding heart disease and stroke.
>
> *(Source: "Diabetes, Heart Disease, and You," Centers for Disease Control and Prevention (CDC).)*

What Else Increases My Chances of Heart Disease or Stroke If I Have Diabetes?

If you have diabetes, other factors add to your chances of developing heart disease or having a stroke.

Smoking

Smoking raises your risk of developing heart disease. If you have diabetes, it is important to stop smoking because both smoking and diabetes narrow blood vessels. Smoking also increases your chances of developing other long-term problems, such as lung disease. Smoking also can damage the blood vessels in your legs and increase the risk of lower leg infections, ulcers, and amputation.

High Blood Pressure

If you have high blood pressure, your heart must work harder to pump blood. High blood pressure can strain your heart; damage blood vessels; and increase your risk of heart attack, stroke, eye problems, and kidney problems.

Abnormal Cholesterol Levels

Cholesterol is a type of fat produced by your liver and found in your blood. You have two kinds of cholesterol in your blood: low-density lipoproteins (LDL) and high-density lipoproteins (HDL).

Low-density lipoprotein, often called "bad cholesterol," can build up and clog your blood vessels. High levels of LDL cholesterol raise your risk of developing heart disease.

Another type of blood fat, triglycerides, also can raise your risk of heart disease when the levels are higher than recommended by your healthcare team.

Obesity and Belly Fat

Being overweight or obese can affect your ability to manage your diabetes and increase your risk for many health problems, including heart disease and high blood pressure. If you are overweight, a healthy eating plan with reduced calories often will lower your glucose levels and reduce your need for medications.

Excess belly fat around your waist, even if you are not overweight, can raise your chances of developing heart disease.

You have excess belly fat if your waist measures:

- More than 40 inches and you are a man
- More than 35 inches and you are a woman

Family History of Heart Disease

A family history of heart disease may also add to your chances of developing heart disease. If one or more of your family members had a heart attack before the age of 50, you may have an even higher chance of developing heart disease.

You cannot change whether heart disease runs in your family, but if you have diabetes, it is even more important to take steps to protect yourself from heart disease and decrease your chances of having a stroke.

How Can I Lower My Chances of a Heart Attack or Stroke If I Have Diabetes?

Taking care of your diabetes is important to help you take care of your heart. You can lower your chances of having a heart attack or stroke by taking the following steps to manage your diabetes to keep your heart and blood vessels healthy.

Manage Your Diabetes ABCs

Knowing your diabetes ABCs will help you manage your blood glucose, blood pressure, and cholesterol. Stopping smoking if you have diabetes is also important to lower your chances for heart disease.

A is for the A1C test. The A1C test shows your average blood glucose level over the past three months. This is different from the blood glucose checks that you do every day. The higher your A1C number, the higher your blood glucose levels have been during the past three months. High levels of blood glucose can harm your heart, blood vessels, kidneys, feet, and eyes.

The A1C goal for many people with diabetes is below seven percent. Some people may do better with a slightly higher A1C goal. Ask your healthcare team what your goal should be.

B is for blood pressure. Blood pressure is the force of your blood against the wall of your blood vessels. If your blood pressure gets too high, it makes your heart work too hard. High blood pressure can cause a heart attack or stroke and damage your kidneys and eyes.

The blood pressure goal for most people with diabetes is below 140/90 mm Hg. Ask what your goal should be.

C is for cholesterol. You have two kinds of cholesterol in your blood: LDL and HDL. LDL can build up and clog your blood vessels. Too much bad cholesterol can cause a heart attack or stroke. HDL or "good" cholesterol helps remove the "bad" cholesterol from your blood vessels.

Ask your healthcare team what your cholesterol numbers should be. If you are over 40 years of age, you may need to take medicine such as a statin to lower your cholesterol and protect your heart. Some people with very high LDL cholesterol may need to take medicine at a younger age.

S is for stop smoking. Not smoking is especially important for people with diabetes because both smoking and diabetes narrow blood vessels, so your heart has to work harder.

If you quit smoking:

- You will lower your risk for heart attack, stroke, nerve disease, kidney disease, eye disease, and amputation.

- Your blood glucose, blood pressure, and cholesterol levels may improve.

- Your blood circulation will improve.

- You may have an easier time being physically active.

If you smoke or use other tobacco products, stop. Ask for help so you do not have to do it alone. You can start by calling the national quitline at 800-QUIT NOW or 800-784-8669.

Ask your healthcare team about your goals for A1C, blood pressure, and cholesterol, and what you can do to reach these goals.

Develop or Maintain Healthy Lifestyle Habits

Developing or maintaining healthy lifestyle habits can help you manage your diabetes and prevent heart disease.

- Follow your healthy eating plan.

- Make physical activity part of your routine.

- Stay at or get to a healthy weight.

- Get enough sleep.

Learn to Manage Stress

Managing diabetes is not always easy. Feeling stressed, sad, or angry is common when you are living with diabetes. You may know what to do to stay healthy but may have trouble sticking with your plan over time. Long-term stress can raise your blood glucose and blood pressure, but you can learn ways to lower your stress. Try deep breathing, gardening, taking a walk, doing yoga, meditating, doing a hobby, or listening to your favorite music.

Take Medicine to Protect Your Heart

Medicines may be an important part of your treatment plan. Your doctor will prescribe medicine based on your specific needs. Medicine may help you:

- Meet your A1C (blood glucose), blood pressure, and cholesterol goals.

- Reduce your risk of blood clots, heart attack, or stroke.

- Treat angina, or chest pain that is often a symptom of heart disease. (Angina can also be an early symptom of a heart attack.)

Ask your doctor whether you should take aspirin. Aspirin is not safe for everyone. Your doctor can tell you whether taking aspirin is right for you and exactly how much to take.

Statins can reduce the risk of having a heart attack or stroke in some people with diabetes. Statins are a type of medicine often used to help people meet their cholesterol goals. Talk with your doctor to find out whether taking a statin is right for you.

Talk with your doctor if you have questions about your medicines. Before you start a new medicine, ask your doctor about possible side effects and how you can avoid them. If the side effects of your medicine bother you, tell your doctor. Do not stop taking your medicines without checking with your doctor first.

How Do Doctors Diagnose Heart Disease in Diabetes?

Doctors diagnose heart disease in diabetes based on:

- Your symptoms

- Your medical and family history

- How likely you are to have heart disease

- A physical exam

- Results from tests and procedures

Tests used to monitor your diabetes—A1C, blood pressure, and cholesterol—help your doctor decide whether it is important to do other tests to check your heart health.

What Are the Warning Signs of Heart Attack and Stroke?

Call 911 right away if you have warning signs of a heart attack:

- Pain or pressure in your chest that lasts longer than a few minutes or goes away and comes back

- Pain or discomfort in one or both of your arms or shoulders; or your back, neck, or jaw

- Shortness of breath

- Sweating or light-headedness

- Indigestion or nausea (feeling sick to your stomach)

- Feeling very tired

Treatment works best when it is given right away. Warning signs can be different in different people. You may not have all of these symptoms.

If you have angina, it is important to know how and when to seek medical treatment.

Women sometimes have nausea and vomiting; feel very tired (sometimes for days); and have pain in the back, shoulders, or jaw without any chest pain.

People with diabetes-related nerve damage may not notice any chest pain.

Call 911 right away if you have warning signs of a stroke, including sudden:

- Weakness or numbness of your face, arm, or leg on one side of your body

- Confusion, or trouble talking or understanding

- Dizziness, loss of balance, or trouble walking

- Trouble seeing out of one or both eyes

- Sudden severe headache

If you have any one of these warning signs, call 911. You can help prevent permanent damage by getting to a hospital within an hour of a stroke.

Chapter 25

Diabetic Neuropathy

What Is Diabetic Neuropathy?

Diabetic neuropathy is nerve damage that is caused by diabetes.

Nerves are bundles of special tissues that carry signals between your brain and other parts of your body. The signals:

- Send information about how things feel
- Move your body parts
- Control body functions, such as digestion

What Are the Different Types of Diabetic Neuropathy?

Types of diabetic neuropathy include the following:

Peripheral Neuropathy

Peripheral neuropathy is nerve damage that typically affects the feet and legs, and sometimes affects the hands and arms.

About This Chapter: This chapter includes text excerpted from "What Is Diabetic Neuropathy?" National Institute of Diabetes and Digestive and Kidney Diseases (NIDDK), February 2018.

Autonomic Neuropathy

Autonomic neuropathy is damage to the nerves that control your internal organs. Autonomic neuropathy can lead to problems with your heart rate and blood pressure, digestive system, bladder, sex organs, sweat glands, eyes, and ability to sense hypoglycemia.

Focal Neuropathies

Focal neuropathies are conditions in which you typically have damage to single nerves, most often in your hand, head, torso, and leg.

Proximal Neuropathy

Proximal neuropathy is a rare and disabling type of nerve damage in your hip, buttock, or thigh. This type of nerve damage typically affects one side of your body and rarely spreads to the other side. Proximal neuropathy often causes severe pain and may lead to significant weight loss.

Who Is Most Likely to Get Diabetic Neuropathy?

If you have diabetes, your chance of developing nerve damage caused by diabetes increases the older you get and the longer you have diabetes. Managing your diabetes is an important part of preventing health problems, such as diabetic neuropathy.

You are also more likely to develop nerve damage if you have diabetes and:

- Are overweight
- Have high blood pressure
- Have high cholesterol
- Have advanced kidney disease
- Drink too many alcoholic drinks
- Smoke

Research also suggests that certain genes may make people more likely to develop diabetic neuropathy.

What Causes Diabetic Neuropathy

Over time, high blood glucose levels, also called "blood sugar," and high levels of fats, such as triglycerides, in the blood from diabetes can damage your nerves. High blood glucose levels can also damage the small blood vessels that nourish your nerves with oxygen and nutrients. Without enough oxygen and nutrients, your nerves cannot function well.

Risk Factors

Nerve damage is likely due to a combination of factors:

- Metabolic factors, such as high blood glucose, long duration of diabetes, abnormal blood fat levels, and possibly low levels of insulin

- Neurovascular factors, leading to damage to the blood vessels that carry oxygen and nutrients to nerves

- Autoimmune factors that cause inflammation in nerves

- Mechanical injury to nerves, such as carpal tunnel syndrome

- Inherited traits that increase susceptibility to nerve disease

- Lifestyle factors, such as smoking or alcohol use

(Source: "Diabetic Neuropathies: The Nerve Damage of Diabetes," Mental Illness Research, Education and Clinical Centers (MIRECC), U.S. Department of Veterans Affairs (VA).)

How Common Is Diabetic Neuropathy?

Although different types of diabetic neuropathy can affect people who have diabetes, research suggests that up to one-half of people with diabetes have peripheral neuropathy. More than 30 percent of people with diabetes have autonomic neuropathy.

The most common type of focal neuropathy is carpal tunnel syndrome (CTS), in which a nerve in your wrist is compressed. Although less than 10 percent of people with diabetes feel symptoms of CTS, about 25 percent of people with diabetes have some nerve compression at the wrist.

Other focal neuropathies and proximal neuropathy are less common.

What Are the Symptoms of Diabetic Neuropathy?

Your symptoms depend on which type of diabetic neuropathy you have. In peripheral neuropathy, some people may have a loss of sensation in their feet, while others may have burning or shooting pain in their lower legs. Most nerve damage develops over many years, and some people may not notice symptoms of mild nerve damage for a long time. In some people, severe pain begins suddenly.

What Problems Does Diabetic Neuropathy Cause?

Peripheral neuropathy can lead to foot complications, such as sores, ulcers, and infections, because nerve damage can make you lose feeling in your feet. As a result, you may not notice that your shoes are causing a sore or that you have injured your feet. Nerve damage can also cause problems with balance and coordination, leading to falls and fractures.

These problems may make it difficult for you to get around easily, causing you to lose some of your independence. In some people with diabetes, nerve damage causes chronic pain, which can lead to anxiety and depression.

Autonomic neuropathy can cause problems with how your organs work, including problems with your heart rate and blood pressure, digestion, urination, and ability to sense when you have low blood glucose.

How Can I Prevent Diabetic Neuropathy?

To prevent diabetic neuropathy, it is important to manage your diabetes by managing your blood glucose, blood pressure, and cholesterol levels.

You should also take the following steps to help prevent diabetes-related nerve damage:

- Be physically active.

- Follow your diabetes meal plan.

- Get help to quit smoking.

- Limit alcoholic drinks to no more than one drink per day for women and no more than two drinks per day for men.

- Take any diabetes medicines and other medicines your doctor prescribes.

How Can I Prevent Diabetic Neuropathy from Getting Worse?

If you have diabetic neuropathy, you should manage your diabetes, which means managing your blood glucose, blood pressure, cholesterol levels, and weight to keep nerve damage from getting worse.

Foot care is very important for all people with diabetes, and it is even more important if you have peripheral neuropathy. Check your feet for problems every day, and take good care of your feet. See your doctor for a neurological exam and a foot exam at least once a year—more often if you have foot problems.

Chapter 26

Diabetic Eye Disease

What Is Diabetic Eye Disease?

Diabetic eye disease is a group of eye problems that can affect people with diabetes. These conditions include diabetic retinopathy, diabetic macular edema, cataracts, and glaucoma.

Over time, diabetes can cause damage to your eyes that can lead to poor vision or even blindness. But, you can take steps to prevent diabetic eye disease, or keep it from getting worse, by taking care of your diabetes.

The best ways to manage your diabetes and keep your eyes healthy are to:

- Manage your blood glucose, blood pressure, and cholesterol; This is sometimes called "the diabetes ABCs."

- If you smoke, get help to quit smoking.

- Have a dilated eye exam once a year.

Often, there are no warning signs of diabetic eye disease or vision loss when damage first develops. A full, dilated eye exam helps your doctor find and treat eye problems early—often before much vision loss can occur.

How Does Diabetes Affect My Eyes?

Diabetes affects your eyes when your blood glucose, also called "blood sugar," is too high.

About This Chapter: This chapter includes text excerpted from "Diabetic Eye Disease," National Institute of Diabetes and Digestive and Kidney Diseases (NIDDK), May 2017.

In the short term, you are not likely to have vision loss from high blood glucose. People sometimes have blurry vision for a few days or weeks when they are changing their diabetes care plan or medicines. High glucose can change fluid levels or cause swelling in the tissues of your eyes that help you to focus, causing blurred vision. This type of blurry vision is temporary and goes away when your glucose level gets closer to normal.

If your blood glucose stays high over time, it can damage the tiny blood vessels in the back of your eyes. This damage can begin during the prediabetes when blood glucose is higher than normal, but it is not yet high enough for you to be diagnosed with diabetes. Damaged blood vessels may leak fluid and cause swelling. New, weak blood vessels may also begin to grow. These blood vessels can bleed into the middle part of the eye, lead to scarring, or cause dangerously high pressure inside your eye.

Most serious diabetic eye diseases begin with blood vessel problems. The four eye diseases that can threaten your sight are:

Diabetic Retinopathy

The retina is the inner lining at the back of each eye. The retina senses light and turns it into signals that your brain decodes, so you can see the world around you. Damaged blood vessels can harm the retina, causing a disease called "diabetic retinopathy."

In early diabetic retinopathy, blood vessels can weaken, bulge, or leak into the retina. This stage is called "nonproliferative diabetic retinopathy."

If the disease gets worse, some blood vessels close off, which causes new blood vessels to grow or proliferate, on the surface of the retina. This stage is called "proliferative diabetic retinopathy." These abnormal new blood vessels can lead to serious vision problems.

Diabetic Macular Edema

The part of your retina that you need for reading, driving, and seeing faces is called the "macula." Diabetes can lead to swelling in the macula, which is called "diabetic macular edema." Over time, this disease can destroy the sharp vision in this part of the eye, leading to partial vision loss or blindness. Macular edema usually develops in people who already have other signs of diabetic retinopathy.

Glaucoma

Glaucoma is a group of eye diseases that can damage the optic nerve—the bundle of nerves that connects the eye to the brain. Diabetes doubles the chances of having glaucoma, which can lead to vision loss and blindness if not treated early.

Cataracts

The lenses within our eyes are clear structures that help provide sharp vision, but they tend to become cloudy as we age. People with diabetes are more likely to develop cloudy lenses, called "cataracts." People with diabetes can develop cataracts at an earlier age than people without diabetes. Researchers think that high glucose levels cause deposits to build up in the lenses of your eyes.

How Common Is Diabetic Eye Disease?
Diabetic Retinopathy

About 1 in 3 people with diabetes who are older than the age of 40 already have some signs of diabetic retinopathy. Diabetic retinopathy is the most common cause of vision loss in people with diabetes. Each person's outlook for the future, however, depends in large part on regular care. Finding and treating diabetic retinopathy early can reduce the risk of blindness by 95 percent.

Glaucoma and Cataracts

Your chances of developing glaucoma or cataracts are about twice that of someone without diabetes.

Who Is More Likely to Develop Diabetic Eye Disease?

Anyone with diabetes can develop diabetic eye disease. Your risk is greater with:

- High blood glucose that is not treated

- High blood pressure that is not treated

High blood cholesterol and smoking may also raise your risk for diabetic eye disease.

Some groups are affected more than others. African Americans, American Indians and Alaska Natives, Hispanics/Latinxs, Pacific Islanders, and older adults are at a greater risk of losing vision or going blind from diabetes.

If you have diabetes and become pregnant, you can develop eye problems very quickly during your pregnancy. If you already have some diabetic retinopathy, it can get worse during pregnancy. Changes that help your body support a fetus may put stress on the blood vessels in your eyes. Your healthcare team will suggest regular eye exams during pregnancy to catch and treat problems early and protect your vision.

Diabetes that occurs only during pregnancy, called "gestational diabetes," does not usually cause eye problems. Researchers are not sure why this is the case.

Your chances of developing diabetic eye disease increase the longer you have diabetes.

What Are the Symptoms of Diabetic Eye Disease?

Often, there are no early symptoms of diabetic eye disease. You may have no pain and no change in your vision as damage begins to grow inside your eyes, particularly with diabetic retinopathy.

When symptoms do occur, they may include:

- Blurry or wavy vision
- Frequently changing vision—sometimes from day to day
- Dark areas or vision loss
- Poor color vision
- Spots or dark strings (also called "floaters")
- Flashes of light

Talk with your eye doctor if you have any of these symptoms.

When Should I See a Doctor?

Call a doctor right away if you notice sudden changes to your vision, including flashes of light or many more spots than usual. You also should see a doctor right away if it looks like a curtain is pulled over your eyes. These changes in your sight can be symptoms of a detached retina, which is a medical emergency.

How Do Doctors Diagnose Eye Problems from Diabetes?

Having a full, dilated eye exam is the best way to check for eye problems from diabetes. Your doctor will place drops in your eyes to widen your pupils. This allows the doctor to examine a larger area at the back of each eye, using a special magnifying lens. Your vision will be blurry for a few hours after a dilated exam.

Your doctor will also:

- Test your vision

- Measure the pressure in your eyes

Your doctor may suggest other tests, too, depending on your health history.

Most people with diabetes should see an eye care professional once a year for a complete eye exam. Your own healthcare team may suggest a different plan, based on your type of diabetes and the time since you were first diagnosed.

How Do Doctors Treat Diabetic Eye Disease?

Your doctor may recommend having eye exams more often than once a year, along with the management of your diabetes. This means managing your diabetes ABCs, which include your A1c, blood pressure, and cholesterol, and quitting smoking. Ask your healthcare team what you can do to reach your goals.

Doctors may treat advanced eye problems with medicine, laser treatments, surgery, or a combination of these options.

Medicine

Your doctor may treat your eyes with anti-vascular endothelial growth factor (VEGF) medicine, such as aflibercept, bevacizumab, or ranibizumab. These medicines block the growth of abnormal blood vessels in the eye. Anti-VEGF medicines can also stop fluid leaks, which can help treat diabetic macular edema.

The doctor will inject an anti-VEGF medicine into your eyes during office visits. You will have several treatments during the first few months, then fewer treatments after you finish the first round of therapy. Your doctor will use medicine to numb your eyes, so you do not feel pain. The needle is about the thickness of a human hair.

Anti-VEGF treatments can stop further vision loss and may improve vision in some people.

Laser Treatment

Laser treatment, also called "photocoagulation," creates tiny burns inside the eye with a beam of light. This method treats leaky blood vessels and extra fluid, called "edema." Your doctor usually provides this treatment during several office visits, using medicine to numb your eyes. Laser treatment can keep eye disease from getting worse, which is important to prevent vision loss or blindness. But, laser treatment is less likely to bring back vision you have already lost when compared with anti-VEGF medicines.

There are two types of laser treatment:

- Focal/grid laser treatment works on a small area of the retina to treat diabetic macular edema.

- Scatter laser treatment, also called "panretinal photocoagulation (PRP)," covers a larger area of the retina. This method treats the growth of abnormal blood vessels, called "proliferative diabetic retinopathy."

Vitrectomy

Vitrectomy is a surgery to remove the clear gel that fills the center of the eye, called the "vitreous gel." The procedure treats problems with severe bleeding or scar tissue caused by proliferative diabetic retinopathy. Scar tissue can force the retina to peel away from the tissue beneath it, similar to wallpaper peeling away from a wall. A retina that comes completely loose, or detaches, can cause blindness.

During a vitrectomy, a clear salt solution is gently pumped into the eye to maintain eye pressure during surgery and to replace the removed vitreous. Vitrectomy is done in a surgery center or hospital with pain medicine.

Cataract Lens Surgery

In a surgery center or hospital visit, your doctor can remove the cloudy lens in your eye, where the cataract has grown, and replace it with an artificial lens. People who have cataract surgery generally have better vision afterward. After your eye heals, you may need a new prescription for your glasses.

What Can I Do to Protect My Eyes?

To prevent diabetic eye disease, or to keep it from getting worse, manage your diabetes ABCs and quit smoking if you smoke.

Also, have a dilated eye exam at least once a year—or more often if recommended by your eye care professional. These actions are powerful ways to protect the health of your eyes—and can prevent blindness.

The sooner you work to manage your diabetes and other health conditions, the better. And, even if you have struggled in the past to manage your health, taking better care of yourself now can protect your eyes for the future. It is never too late to begin.

What If I Already Have Some Vision Loss from Diabetes?

Ask your eye care professional to help you find a low vision and rehabilitation clinic. Special eye care professionals can help you manage vision loss that cannot be corrected with glasses, contact lenses, medicine, or surgery. Special devices and training may help you make the most of your remaining vision so that you can continue to be active, enjoy hobbies, visit friends and family members, and live without help from others.

Chapter 27

Diabetic Kidney Disease

What Is Diabetic Kidney Disease?

Diabetic kidney disease is a type of kidney disease caused by diabetes.

Diabetes is the leading cause of kidney disease. About one out of four adults with diabetes has kidney disease.

The main job of the kidneys is to filter wastes and extra water out of your blood to make urine. Your kidneys also help control blood pressure and make hormones that your body needs to stay healthy.

When your kidneys are damaged, they cannot filter blood like they should, which can cause wastes to build up in your body. Kidney damage can also cause other health problems.

Kidney damage caused by diabetes usually occurs slowly, over many years. You can take steps to protect your kidneys and to prevent or delay kidney damage.

What Are Other Names for Diabetic Kidney Disease?
Diabetic kidney disease is also called "DKD," "chronic kidney disease" (CKD), "kidney disease of diabetes," or "diabetic nephropathy."

About This Chapter: This chapter includes text excerpted from "Diabetic Kidney Disease," National Institute of Diabetes and Digestive and Kidney Diseases (NIDDK), February 2017.

How Does Diabetes Cause Kidney Disease?

High blood glucose, also called "blood sugar," can damage the blood vessels in your kidneys. When the blood vessels are damaged, they do not work as well. Many people with diabetes also develop high blood pressure, which can also damage your kidneys.

What Increases My Chances of Developing Diabetic Kidney Disease?

Having diabetes for a longer time increases the chances that you will have kidney damage. If you have diabetes, you are more likely to develop kidney disease if your:

- Blood glucose is too high
- Blood pressure is too high

African Americans, American Indians, and Hispanics/Latinxs develop diabetes, kidney disease, and kidney failure at a higher rate than Caucasians.

You are also more likely to develop kidney disease if you have diabetes and:

- Smoke
- Do not follow your diabetes eating plan
- Eat foods high in salt
- Are not active
- Are overweight
- Have heart disease
- Have a family history of kidney failure

How Can I Tell If I Have Diabetic Kidney Disease?

Most people with diabetic kidney disease do not have symptoms. The only way to know if you have diabetic kidney disease is to get your kidneys checked.

Healthcare professionals use blood and urine tests to check for diabetic kidney disease. Your healthcare professional will check your urine for albumin and will also do a blood test to see how well your kidneys are filtering your blood.

You should get tested every year for kidney disease if you:

- Have type 2 diabetes
- Have had type 1 diabetes for more than five years

How Can I Keep My Kidneys Healthy If I Have Diabetes?

The best way to slow or prevent diabetes-related kidney disease is to try to reach your blood glucose and blood pressure goals. Healthy lifestyle habits and taking your medicines as prescribed can help you achieve these goals and improve your overall health.

Reach Your Blood Glucose Goals

Your healthcare professional will test your A1C. The A1C is a blood test that shows your average blood glucose level over the past three months. This is different from the blood glucose checks that you may do yourself. The higher your A1C number, the higher your blood glucose levels have been during the past three months.

The A1C goal for many people with diabetes is below seven percent. Ask your healthcare team what your goal should be. Reaching your goal numbers will help you protect your kidneys.

To reach your A1C goal, your healthcare professional may ask you to check your blood glucose levels. Work with your healthcare team to use the results to guide decisions about food, physical activity, and medicines. Ask your healthcare team how often you should check your blood glucose level.

Control Your Blood Pressure

Blood pressure is the force of your blood against the wall of your blood vessels. High blood pressure makes your heart work too hard. It can cause a heart attack, stroke, and kidney disease.

Your healthcare team will also work with you to help you set and reach your blood pressure goal. The blood pressure goal for most people with diabetes is below 140/90 mm Hg. Ask your healthcare team what your goal should be.

Medicines that lower blood pressure can also help slow kidney damage. Two types of blood pressure medicines, angiotensin-converting-enzyme (ACE) inhibitors and angiotensin II receptor blockers (ARBs), play a special role in protecting your kidneys. Each has been found to slow kidney damage in people with diabetes who have high blood pressure and DKD. The names of these medicines end in -pril or -sartan. ACE inhibitors and ARBs are not safe for women who are pregnant.

Develop or Maintain Healthy Lifestyle Habits

Healthy lifestyle habits can help you reach your blood glucose and blood pressure goals. Following the steps below will also help you keep your kidneys healthy:

- Stop smoking.
- Work with a dietitian to develop a diabetes meal plan and limit salt and sodium.
- Make physical activity part of your routine.
- Stay at or get to a healthy weight.
- Get enough sleep. Aim for seven to eight hours of sleep each night.

Take Medicines as Prescribed

Medicines may be an important part of your treatment plan. Your healthcare professional will prescribe medicine based on your specific needs. Medicine can help you meet your blood glucose and blood pressure goals. You may need to take more than one kind of medicine to control your blood pressure.

How Can I Cope with the Stress of Managing My Diabetes?

Managing diabetes is not always easy. Feeling stressed, sad, or angry is common when you are living with diabetes. You may know what to do to stay healthy but may have trouble sticking with your plan over time. Long-term stress can raise your blood glucose and blood pressure, but you can learn ways to lower your stress. Try deep breathing, gardening, taking a walk, doing yoga, meditating, doing a hobby, or listening to your favorite music.

Does Diabetic Kidney Disease Get Worse Over Time?

Kidney damage from diabetes can get worse over time. However, you can take steps to keep your kidneys healthy and help slow kidney damage to prevent or delay kidney failure.

Kidney failure means that your kidneys have lost most of their ability to function—less than 15 percent of normal kidney function. However, most people with diabetes and kidney disease do not end up with kidney failure.

Chapter 28

Gastroparesis

What Is Gastroparesis?

Gastroparesis, also called "delayed gastric emptying," is a disorder that slows or stops the movement of food from your stomach to your small intestine. Normally, after you swallow food, the muscles in the wall of your stomach grind the food into smaller pieces and push them into your small intestine to continue digestion. When you have gastroparesis, your stomach muscles work poorly or not at all, and your stomach takes too long to empty its contents. Gastroparesis can delay digestion, which can lead to various symptoms and complications.

How Common Is Gastroparesis?

Gastroparesis is not common. Out of 100,000 people, about 10 men and about 40 women have gastroparesis. However, symptoms that are similar to those of gastroparesis occur in about 1 out of 4 adults in the United States.

About This Chapter: Text beginning with the heading "What Is Gastroparesis?" is excerpted from "Definition and Facts for Gastroparesis," National Institute of Diabetes and Digestive and Kidney Diseases (NIDDK), January 2018; Text beginning with the heading "How Do Doctors Treat Gastroparesis?" is excerpted from "Treatment for Gastroparesis," National Institute of Diabetes and Digestive and Kidney Diseases (NIDDK), January 2018; Text beginning with the heading "How Can My Diet Help Prevent or Relieve Gastroparesis?" is excerpted from "Eating, Diet, and Nutrition for Gastroparesis," National Institute of Diabetes and Digestive and Kidney Diseases (NIDDK), January 2018.

Who Is More Likely to Get Gastroparesis?

You are more likely to get gastroparesis if you:

- Have diabetes

- Had surgery on your esophagus, stomach, or small intestine, which may injure the vagus nerve. The vagus nerve controls the muscles of the stomach and small intestine.

- Had certain cancer treatments, such as radiation therapy on your chest or stomach area

What Other Health Problems Do People with Gastroparesis Have?

People with gastroparesis may have other health problems, such as:

- Diabetes

- Scleroderma

- Hypothyroidism

- Nervous system disorders, such as migraine, Parkinson disease (PD), and multiple sclerosis (MS)

- Gastroesophageal reflux disease (GERD)

- Eating disorders

- Amyloidosis

What Are the Complications of Gastroparesis?

Complications of gastroparesis may include:

- Blood glucose, also called "blood sugar," levels that are harder to control, which can worsen diabetes

- Dehydration due to repeated vomiting

- Malnutrition due to poor absorption of nutrients

- Low-calorie intake

- Bezoars

- Losing weight without trying

- Lower quality of life (QOL)

How Do Doctors Treat Gastroparesis?

How doctors treat gastroparesis depends on the cause, how severe your symptoms and complications are, and how well you respond to different treatments. Sometimes, treating the cause may stop gastroparesis. If diabetes is causing your gastroparesis, your healthcare professional will work with you to help control your blood glucose levels. When the cause of your gastroparesis is not known, your doctor will provide treatments to help relieve your symptoms and treat complications.

Changing Eating Habits

Changing your eating habits can help control gastroparesis and make sure you get the right amount of nutrients, calories, and liquids. Getting the right amount of nutrients, calories, and liquids can also treat the disorder two main complications: malnutrition and dehydration.

Your doctor may recommend that you:

- Eat foods low in fat and fiber.
- Eat five or six small, nutritious meals a day instead of two or three large meals.
- Chew your food thoroughly.
- Eat soft, well-cooked food.
- Avoid carbonated, or fizzy, beverages.
- Avoid alcohol.
- Drink plenty of water or liquids that contain glucose and electrolytes, such as:
  - Low-fat broths or clear soups
  - Naturally sweetened, low-fiber fruit, and vegetable juices
  - Sports drinks
  - Oral rehydration solutions
- Do some gentle physical activity after a meal, such as taking a walk.
- Avoid lying down for two hours after a meal.
- Take a multivitamin each day.

If your symptoms are moderate to severe, your doctor may recommend drinking only liquids or eating well-cooked solid foods that have been processed into very small pieces or paste in a blender.

Controlling Blood Glucose Levels

If you have gastroparesis and diabetes, you will need to control your blood glucose levels, especially hyperglycemia. Hyperglycemia may further delay the emptying of food from your stomach. Your doctor will work with you to make sure your blood glucose levels are not too high or too low and do not keep going up or down. Your doctor may recommend:

- Taking insulin more often, or changing the type of insulin you take

- Taking insulin after, instead of before, meals

- Checking your blood glucose levels often after you eat, and taking insulin when you need it

Your doctor will give you specific instructions for taking insulin based on your needs and the severity of your gastroparesis.

Medicines

Your doctor may prescribe medicines that help the muscles in the wall of your stomach work better. She or he may also prescribe medicines to control nausea and vomiting and reduce pain.

Your doctor may prescribe one or more of the following medicines:

- **Metoclopramide.** This medicine increases the tightening, or contraction, of the muscles in the wall of your stomach and may improve gastric emptying. Metoclopramide may also help relieve nausea and vomiting.

- **Domperidone.** This medicine also increases the contraction of the muscles in the wall of your stomach and may improve gastric emptying. However, this medicine is available for use only under a special program administered by the U.S. Food and Drug Administration (FDA).

- **Erythromycin.** This medicine also increases stomach muscle contraction and may improve gastric emptying.

- **Antiemetics.** Antiemetics are medicines that help relieve nausea and vomiting. Prescription antiemetics include ondansetron, prochlorperazine, and promethazine. Over-the-counter (OTC) antiemetics include bismuth subsalicylate and diphenhydramine. Antiemetics do not improve gastric emptying.

- **Antidepressants.** Certain antidepressants, such as mirtazapine, may help relieve nausea and vomiting. These medicines may not improve gastric emptying.

- **Pain medicines.** Pain medicines that are not narcotic pain medicines may reduce pain in your abdomen due to gastroparesis.

Oral or Nasal Tube Feeding

In some cases, your doctor may recommend oral or nasal tube feeding to make sure you are getting the right amount of nutrients and calories. A healthcare professional will put a tube either into your mouth or nose, through your esophagus and stomach, to your small intestine. Oral and nasal tube feeding bypass your stomach and deliver a special liquid food directly into your small intestine.

Jejunostomy Tube Feeding

If you are not getting enough nutrients and calories from other treatments, your doctor may recommend jejunostomy tube feeding. Jejunostomy feedings are a longer term method of feeding, compared to oral or nasal tube feeding.

Jejunostomy tube feeding is a way to feed you through a tube placed into part of your small intestine called the "jejunum." To place the tube into the jejunum, a doctor creates an opening, called a "jejunostomy," in your abdominal wall that goes into your jejunum. The feeding tube bypasses your stomach and delivers a liquid food directly into your jejunum.

Parenteral Nutrition

Your doctor may recommend parenteral, or intravenous (IV), nutrition if your gastroparesis is so severe that other treatments are not helping. Parenteral nutrition delivers liquid nutrients directly into your bloodstream. Parenteral nutrition may be short term, until you can eat again. Parenteral nutrition may also be used until a tube can be placed for oral, nasal, or jejunostomy tube feeding. In some cases, parenteral nutrition may be long-term.

Venting Gastrostomy

Your doctor may recommend a venting gastrostomy to relieve pressure inside your stomach. A doctor creates an opening, called a "gastrostomy," in your abdominal wall and into your stomach. The doctor then places a tube through the gastrostomy into your stomach. Stomach contents can then flow out of the tube and relieve pressure inside your stomach.

Gastric Electrical Stimulation

Gastric electrical stimulation (GES) uses a small, battery-powered device to send mild electrical pulses to the nerves and muscles in the lower stomach. A surgeon puts the device under the skin in your lower abdomen and attaches wires from the device to the muscles in the wall of your stomach. GES can help decrease long-term nausea and vomiting.

Gastric electrical stimulation is used to treat people with gastroparesis due to diabetes or unknown causes only, and only in people whose symptoms cannot be controlled with medicines.

How Can I Prevent Gastroparesis?

Gastroparesis without a known cause, called "idiopathic gastroparesis," cannot be prevented.

If you have diabetes, you can prevent or delay nerve damage that can cause gastroparesis by keeping your blood glucose levels within the target range that your doctor thinks is best for you. Meal planning, physical activity, and medicines, if needed, can help you keep your blood glucose levels within your target range.

How Can My Diet Help Prevent or Relieve Gastroparesis?

What you eat can help prevent or relieve your gastroparesis symptoms. If you have diabetes, following a healthy meal plan can help you manage your blood glucose levels. What you eat can also help make sure you get the right amount of nutrients, calories, and liquids if you are malnourished or dehydrated from gastroparesis.

What Should I Eat and Drink If I Have Gastroparesis?

If you have gastroparesis, your doctor may recommend that you eat or drink:

- Foods and beverages that are low in fat
- Foods and beverages that are low in fiber
- Five or six small, nutritious meals a day instead of two or three large meals
- Soft, well-cooked foods

If you are unable to eat solid foods, your doctor may recommend that you drink:

- Liquid nutrition meals

- Solid foods puréed in a blender

Your doctor may also recommend that you drink plenty of water or liquids that contain glucose and electrolytes, such as:

- Low-fat broths and clear soups

- Low-fiber fruit and vegetable juices

- Sports drinks

- Oral rehydration solutions

If your symptoms are moderate to severe, your doctor may recommend drinking only liquids or eating well-cooked solid foods that have been processed into very small pieces or paste in a blender.

What Should I Avoid Eating and Drinking If I Have Gastroparesis?

If you have gastroparesis, you should avoid:

- Foods and beverages that are high in fat

- Foods and beverages that are high in fiber

- Foods that cannot be chewed easily

- Carbonated, or fizzy, beverages

- Alcohol

Your doctor may refer you to a dietitian to help you plan healthy meals that are easy for you to digest and give you the right amount of nutrients, calories, and liquids.

Chapter 29

Tooth and Gum Problems Caused by Diabetes

How Can Diabetes Affect My Mouth?

Too much glucose, also called "sugar," in your blood from diabetes can cause pain, infection, and other problems in your mouth. Your mouth includes:

- Your teeth

- Your gums

- Your jaw

- Tissues, such as your tongue, the roof, and bottom of your mouth, and the inside of your cheeks

Glucose is present in your saliva—the fluid in your mouth that makes it wet. When diabetes is not controlled, high glucose levels in your saliva help harmful bacteria grow. These bacteria combine with food to form a soft, sticky film called "plaque." Plaque also comes from eating foods that contain sugars or starches. Some types of plaque cause tooth decay or cavities. Other types of plaque cause gum disease and bad breath.

Gum disease can be more severe and take longer to heal if you have diabetes. In turn, having gum disease can make your blood glucose hard to control.

About This Chapter: This chapter includes text excerpted from "Diabetes, Gum Disease and Other Dental Problems," National Institute of Diabetes and Digestive and Kidney Diseases (NIDDK), September 2014. Reviewed June 2019.

Some people with diabetes really do have a sweet tooth—or rather, a whole mouthful of them. If the sugar level is high in your blood, it's high in your saliva too, which is a problem because sugar serves as a kind of fertilizer for all the bacteria in the mouth. Combined with food, bacteria creates plaque, a sticky film that can cause tooth decay.

And let's not sugar-coat it—diabetes is associated with gum disease, and gum disease can lead to tooth loss and make blood sugar rise, making diabetes harder to control. Gum disease itself can even increase the risk of type 2 diabetes.

But, this will help put the smile back on your face: Treating gum disease in people with type 2 diabetes can lower blood sugar over time and reduce the chance of developing other problems related to diabetes, such as heart and kidney disease.

(Source: "Diabetes and Your Smile," Centers for Disease Control and Prevention (CDC).)

What Happens If I Have Plaque

Plaque that is not removed hardens over time into tartar and collects above your gum line. Tartar makes it more difficult to brush and clean between your teeth. Your gums become red and swollen, and they bleed easily—signs of unhealthy or inflamed gums, called "gingivitis."

When gingivitis is not treated, it can advance to gum disease called "periodontitis." In periodontitis, the gums pull away from the teeth and form spaces, called "pockets," which slowly become infected. This infection can last a long time. Your body fights the bacteria as the plaque spreads and grows below the gum line. Both the bacteria and your body's response to this infection start to break down the bone and the tissue that holds the teeth in place. If periodontitis is not treated, the gums, bones, and tissue that support the teeth are destroyed. Teeth may become loose and might need to be removed. If you have periodontitis, your dentist may send you to a periodontist, an expert in treating gum disease.

What Are the Most Common Mouth Problems from Diabetes?

Few symptoms of a problem in your mouth are sore/ulcer; holes in your teeth; pain in mouth, face, or jaw; loose teeth; pain while chewing; changed sense of taste or a bad taste; and bad breath.

The main symptoms are listed out in the following table.

Table 29.1. Most Common Mouth Problems from Diabetes

Problem	What It Is	Symptoms	Treatment
Gingivitis	Unhealthy or inflamed gums	Red, swollen, and bleeding gums	• Daily brushing and flossing • Regular cleanings at the dentist
Periodontitis	Gum disease, which can change from mild to severe	• Red, swollen, and bleeding gums • Gums that have pulled away from the teeth • Long-lasting infection between the teeth and gums • Bad breath that won't go away • Permanent teeth that are loose or moving away from one another • Changes in the way your teeth fit together when you bite • Sometimes pus between the teeth and gums • Changes in the fit of dentures, which are teeth you can remove	• Deep cleaning at your dentist • Medicine that your dentist prescribes • Gum surgery in severe cases
Thrush, called candidiasis	The growth of a naturally occurring fungus that the body is unable to control	• Sore, white—or sometimes red—patches on your gums, tongue, cheeks, or the roof of your mouth • Patches that have turned into open sores	• Medicine that your doctor or dentist prescribes to kill the fungus • Cleaning dentures • Removing dentures for part of the day or night, and soaking them in medicine that your doctor or dentist prescribes

Table 29.1. Continued

Problem	What It Is	Symptoms	Treatment
Dry mouth, called xerostomia	A lack of saliva in your mouth, which raises your risk for tooth decay and gum disease	• Dry feeling in your mouth, often or all of the time • Dry, rough tongue • Pain in the mouth • Cracked lips • Mouth sores or infection • Problems chewing, eating, swallowing, or talking	• Taking medicine to keep your mouth wet that your doctor or dentist prescribes • Rinsing with a fluoride mouth rinse to prevent cavities • Using sugarless gum or mints to increase saliva flow • Taking frequent sips of water • Avoiding tobacco, caffeine, and alcoholic beverages • Using a humidifier, a device that raises the level of moisture in your home, at night • Avoiding spicy or salty foods that may cause pain in a dry mouth
Oral burning	A burning sensation inside the mouth caused by uncontrolled blood glucose levels	• Burning feeling in the mouth • Dry mouth • Bitter taste • Symptoms may worsen throughout the day	• Seeing your doctor, who may change your diabetes medicine • Once your blood glucose is under control, the oral burning will go away

How Will I Know If I Have Mouth Problems from Diabetes?

Check your mouth for signs of problems from diabetes. If you notice any problems, see your dentist right away. Some of the first signs of gum disease are swollen, tender, or bleeding gums. Sometimes, you would not have any signs of gum disease. You may not know you have it until you have serious damage. Your best defense is to see your dentist twice a year for a cleaning and checkup.

How Can I Prepare for a Visit to My Dentist?

Plan ahead. Talk with your doctor and dentist before the visit about the best way to take care of your blood glucose during dental work.

You may be taking a diabetes medicine that can cause low blood glucose, also called "hypoglycemia." If you take insulin or other diabetes medicines, take them and eat as usual before visiting the dentist. You may need to bring your diabetes medicines and your snacks or meal with you to the dentist's office.

You may need to postpone any nonemergency dental work if your blood glucose is not under control.

If you feel nervous about visiting the dentist, tell your dentist and the staff about your feelings. Your dentist can adapt the treatment to your needs. Do not let your nerves stop you from having regular checkups. Waiting too long to take care of your mouth may make things worse.

What If My Mouth Is Sore after My Dental Work?

A sore mouth is common after dental work. If this happens, you might not be able to eat or chew the foods you normally eat for several hours or days. For guidance on how to adjust your usual routine while your mouth is healing, ask your doctor:

- What foods and drinks you should have

- If you should change the time when you take your diabetes medicines

- If you should change the dose of your diabetes medicines

- How often you should check your blood glucose

How Does Smoking Affect My Mouth?

Smoking makes problems with your mouth worse. Smoking raises your chances of getting gum disease, oral and throat cancers, and oral fungal infections. Smoking also discolors your teeth and makes your breath smell bad.

Smoking and diabetes are a dangerous mix. Smoking raises your risk for many diabetes problems. If you quit smoking:

- You will lower your risk for heart attack, stroke, nerve disease, kidney disease, and amputation

- Your cholesterol and blood pressure levels might improve.

- Your blood circulation will improve.

If you smoke, stop smoking. Ask for help so that you do not have to do it alone. You can start by calling 800-QUIT-NOW or 800-784-8669.

How Can I Keep My Mouth Healthy?

You can keep your mouth healthy by taking these steps:

- Keep your blood glucose numbers as close to your target as possible. Your doctor will help you set your target blood glucose numbers and teach you what to do if your numbers are too high or too low.

- Eat healthy meals and follow the meal plan that you and your doctor or dietitian have worked out.

- Brush your teeth at least twice a day with fluoride toothpaste. Fluoride protects against tooth decay.

  - Aim for brushing first thing in the morning, before going to bed, and after each meal and sugary or starchy snack.

  - Use a soft toothbrush.

  - Gently brush your teeth with the toothbrush angled towards the gum line.

  - Use small, circular motions.

  - Brush the front, back, and top of each tooth. Brush your tongue too.

- Change your toothbrush every three months or sooner if the toothbrush looks worn or the bristles spread out. A new toothbrush removes more plaque.

- Drink water that contains added fluoride or ask your dentist about using a fluoride mouth rinse to prevent tooth decay.

- Ask your dentist about using an antiplaque or antigingivitis mouth rinse to control plaque or prevent gum disease.

- Use dental floss to clean between your teeth at least once a day. Flossing helps prevent plaque from building up on your teeth. When flossing:

  - Slide the floss up and down and then curve it around the base of each tooth under the gums.

  - Use clean sections of floss as you move from tooth to tooth.

- Another way of removing plaque between teeth is to use a dental pick or brush—thin tools designed to clean between the teeth. You can buy these picks at drug stores or grocery stores.

- If you wear dentures, keep them clean and take them out at night. Have them adjusted if they become loose or uncomfortable.

- Call your dentist right away if you have any symptoms of mouth problems.

- See your dentist twice a year for a cleaning and checkup. Your dentist may suggest more visits if you need them.

- Follow your dentist's advice.

  - If your dentist tells you about a problem, take care of it right away.

  - Follow any steps or treatments from your dentist to keep your mouth healthy.

- Tell your dentist that you have diabetes.

  - Tell your dentist about any changes in your health or medicines.

  - Share the results of some of your diabetes blood tests, such as the A1C test or the fasting blood glucose test.

  - Ask if you need antibiotics before and after dental treatment if your diabetes is uncontrolled.

- If you smoke, stop smoking.

Chapter 30

Foot and Skin Problems Caused by Diabetes

Foot problems are common in people with diabetes. You might be afraid you will lose a toe, foot, or leg to diabetes, or know someone who has, but you can lower your chances of having diabetes-related foot problems by taking care of your feet every day. Managing your blood glucose levels, also called "blood sugar," can also help keep your feet healthy

How Can Diabetes Affect My Feet?

Over time, diabetes may cause nerve damage, also called "diabetic neuropathy," that can cause tingling and pain, and can make you lose feeling in your feet. When you lose feeling in your feet, you may not feel a pebble inside your sock or a blister on your foot, which can lead to cuts and sores. Cuts and sores can become infected.

Diabetes also can lower the amount of blood flow in your feet. Not having enough blood flowing to your legs and feet can make it hard for a sore or an infection to heal. Sometimes, a bad infection never heals. The infection might lead to gangrene.

Gangrene and foot ulcers that do not get better with treatment can lead to an amputation of your toe, foot, or part of your leg. A surgeon may perform an amputation to prevent a bad infection from spreading to the rest of your body and to save your life. Good foot care is very important to prevent serious infections and gangrene.

About This Chapter: Text in this chapter begins with excerpts from "Diabetes and Foot Problems," National Institute of Diabetes and Digestive and Kidney Diseases (NIDDK), January 2017; Text beginning with the heading "How Can Diabetes Hurt My Skin?" is excerpted from "Prevent Diabetes Problems: Keep Your Feet and Skin Healthy," National Institute of Diabetes and Digestive and Kidney Diseases (NIDDK), May 2008. Reviewed June 2019.

Although rare, nerve damage from diabetes can lead to changes in the shape of your feet, such as Charcot's foot. Charcot's foot may start with redness, warmth, and swelling. Later, bones in your feet and toes can shift or break, which can cause your feet to have an odd shape, such as a "rocker bottom."

What Can I Do to Keep My Feet Healthy?

Work with your healthcare team to make a diabetes self-care plan, which is an action plan for how you will manage your diabetes. Your plan should include foot care. A foot doctor, also called a "podiatrist," and other specialists may be part of your healthcare team.

Include these steps in your foot care plan.

Check Your Feet Every Day

You may have foot problems but feel no pain in your feet. Checking your feet each day will help you spot problems early before they get worse. A good way to remember is to check your feet each evening when you take off your shoes. Also, check between your toes. If you have trouble bending over to see your feet, try using a mirror to see them, or ask someone else to look at your feet.

Look for problems such as:

- Cuts, sores, or red spots

- Swelling or fluid-filled blisters

- Ingrown toenails, in which the edge of your nail grows into your skin

- Corns or calluses, which are spots of rough skin caused by too much rubbing or pressure on the same spot

- Plantar warts, which are flesh-colored growths on the bottom of the feet

- Athlete's foot

- Warm spots

If you have certain foot problems that make it more likely you will develop a sore on your foot, your doctor may recommend taking the temperature of the skin on different parts of your feet. A "hot spot" can be the first sign that a blister or an ulcer is starting.

Cover a blister, cut, or sore with a bandage. Smooth corns and calluses as explained below.

Wash Your Feet Every Day

Wash your feet with soap in warm, not hot, water. Test the water to make sure it is not too hot. You can use a thermometer (90° to 95°F is safe) or your elbow to test the warmth of the water. Do not soak your feet because your skin will get too dry.

After washing and drying your feet, put talcum powder or cornstarch between your toes. Skin between the toes tends to stay moist. The powder will keep the skin dry to help prevent an infection.

Smooth Corns and Calluses Gently

Thick patches of skin called "corns" or "calluses" can grow on the feet. If you have corns or calluses, talk with your foot doctor about the best way to care for these foot problems. If you have nerve damage, these patches can become ulcers.

If your doctor tells you to, use a pumice stone to smooth corns and calluses after bathing or showering. A pumice stone is a type of rock used to smooth the skin. Rub gently, only in one direction, to avoid tearing the skin.

Do not:

- Cut corns and calluses.

- Use corn plasters, which are medicated pads.

- Use liquid corn and callus removers.

Cutting and over the counter (OTC) corn removal products can damage your skin and cause an infection.

To keep your skin smooth and soft, rub a thin coat of lotion, cream, or petroleum jelly on the tops and bottoms of your feet. Do not put lotion or cream between your toes because moistness might cause an infection.

Trim Your Toenails Straight Across

Trim your toenails, when needed, after you wash and dry your feet. Using toenail clippers, trim your toenails straight across. Do not cut into the corners of your toenail. Gently smooth each nail with an emery board or nonsharp nail file. Trimming this way helps prevent cutting your skin and keeps the nails from growing into your skin.

Have a foot doctor trim your toenails if:

- You cannot see, feel, or reach your feet

- Your toenails are thick or yellowed

- Your nails curve and grow into the skin

If you want to get a pedicure at a salon, you should bring your own nail tools to prevent getting an infection. You can ask your healthcare provider what other steps you can take at the salon to prevent infection.

Wear Shoes and Socks at All Times

Wear shoes and socks at all times. Do not walk barefoot or in just socks—even when you are indoors. You could step on something and hurt your feet. You may not feel any pain and may not know that you hurt yourself.

Check the inside of your shoes before putting them on to make sure the lining is smooth and free of pebbles or other objects.

Make sure you wear socks, stockings, or nylons with your shoes to keep from getting blisters and sores. Choose clean, lightly padded socks that fit well. Socks with no seams are best.

Wear shoes that fit well and protect your feet. Here are some tips for finding the right type of shoes:

- Walking shoes and athletic shoes are good for daily wear. They support your feet and allow them to "breathe."

- Do not wear vinyl or plastic shoes because they do not stretch or "breathe."

- When buying shoes, make sure they feel good and have enough room for your toes. Buy shoes at the end of the day, when your feet are the largest, so that you can find the best fit.

- If you have a bunion, or hammertoes, which are toes that curl under your feet, you may need extra-wide or deep shoes. Do not wear shoes with pointed toes or high heels, because they put too much pressure on your toes.

- If your feet have changed shape, such as from Charcot's foot, you may need special shoes or shoe inserts, called "orthotics." You also may need inserts if you have bunions, hammertoes, or other foot problems.

When breaking in new shoes, only wear them for a few hours at first and then check your feet for areas of soreness.

Medicare Part B insurance and other health insurance programs may help pay for these special shoes or inserts. Ask your insurance plan if it covers your special shoes or inserts.

Protect Your Feet from Hot and Cold

If you have nerve damage from diabetes, you may burn your feet and not know you did. Take the following steps to protect your feet from heat:

- Wear shoes at the beach and on hot pavement.
- Put sunscreen on the tops of your feet to prevent sunburn.
- Keep your feet away from heaters and open fires.
- Do not put a hot water bottle or heating pad on your feet.

Wear socks in bed if your feet get cold. In the winter, wear lined, waterproof boots to keep your feet warm and dry.

Keep the Blood Flowing to Your Feet

Try the following tips to improve blood flow to your feet:

- Put your feet up when you are sitting.
- Wiggle your toes for a few minutes throughout the day. Move your ankles up and down and in and out to help blood flow in your feet and legs.
- Do not wear tight socks or elastic stockings. Do not try to hold up loose socks with rubber bands.
- Be more physically active. Choose activities that are easy on your feet, such as walking, dancing, yoga or stretching, swimming, or bike riding.
- Stop smoking.

Smoking can lower the amount of blood flow to your feet. If you smoke, ask for help to stop. You can get help by calling the national quitline at 800-QUITNOW or 800-784-8669.

Get a Foot Check at Every Healthcare Visit

Ask your healthcare team to check your feet at each visit. Take off your shoes and socks when you are in the exam room so they will remember to check your feet. At least once a year, get a thorough foot exam, including a check of the feeling and pulses in your feet.

Get a thorough foot exam at each healthcare visit if you have:

- Changes in the shape of your feet
- Loss of feeling in your feet

- Peripheral artery disease

- Had foot ulcers or an amputation in the past

Ask your healthcare team to show you how to care for your feet.

Questions to Ask
- Do I inspect my feet daily for wounds or infection?
- Do I wash and care for my feet and skin properly?
- Does my doctor examine my feet each time I visit?
- Do I choose the right shoes?
- Is there anything that I can do to improve my diabetes control?

(Source: "Diabetes Foot and Skin Care," Centers for Disease Control and Prevention (CDC).)

When Should I See My Healthcare Provider about Foot Problems?

Call your healthcare provider right away if you have:

- A cut, blister, or bruise on your foot that does not start to heal after a few days

- Skin on your foot that becomes red, warm, or painful—signs of a possible infection

- A callus with dried blood inside of it, which often can be the first sign of a wound under the callus

- A foot infection that becomes black and smelly—signs you might have gangrene

Ask your provider to refer you to a foot doctor, or podiatrist, if needed.

How Can Diabetes Hurt My Skin?

Diabetes can hurt your skin in two ways:

- If your blood glucose is high, your body loses fluid. With less fluid in your body, your skin can get dry. Dry skin can be itchy, causing you to scratch and make it sore. Also, dry skin can crack. Cracks allow germs to enter and cause infection. If your blood glucose is high, it feeds germs and makes infections worse. You may get dry skin on your legs, feet, elbows, and other places on your body.

- Nerve damage can decrease the amount you sweat. Sweating helps keep your skin soft and moist. Decreased sweating in your feet and legs can cause dry skin.

What Can I Do to Take Care of My Skin?

- After you wash with a mild soap, make sure you rinse and dry yourself well. Check places where water can hide, such as under the arms, under the breasts, between the legs, and between the toes.

- Keep your skin moist by using a lotion or cream after you wash. Ask your doctor to suggest one.

- Drink lots of fluids, such as water, to keep your skin moist and healthy.

- Wear all-cotton underwear. Cotton allows air to move around your body better.

- Check your skin after you wash. Make sure you have no dry, red, or sore spots that might lead to an infection.

- Tell your doctor about any skin problems.

Chapter 31

Acanthosis Nigricans and Necrobiosis Lipoidica

Acanthosis Nigricans

Acanthosis nigricans (AN) is a skin disorder in which there is darker, thick, velvety skin in body folds and creases. This condition usually appears slowly and does not cause any symptoms other than skin changes. Eventually, dark, velvety skin with very visible markings and creases appears in the armpits, groin and neck folds, and over the joints of the fingers and toes. Less commonly, the lips, palms, soles of the feet, or other areas may be affected. The exact cause of this condition is not well understood; but it can be inherited or related to medical problems, such as obesity, diabetes mellitus (insulin-resistance), some prescription drugs, and cancer.

Treatment of Acanthosis Nigricans

There is no specific treatment for AN. Treatments are used mostly to improve cosmetic appearance and include topical retinoids, vitamin D creams (such as calcipotriol), dermabrasion, and laser therapy. Oral retinoid pills have also been used to treat AN, but they are not used for most patients because of the multiple side effects and development problems associated with the treatment. Treatment may also focus on trying to correct the underlying disease that causes AN to develop. Often correcting the underlying disease improves the skin symptoms. Some steps that can be taken depending on the underlying disease include correcting

About This Chapter: Text under the heading "Acanthosis Nigricans" is excerpted from "Acanthosis Nigricans," Genetic and Rare Diseases Information Center (GARD), National Center for Advancing Translational Sciences (NCATS), August 18, 2014. Reviewed June 2019; Text under the heading "Necrobiosis Lipoidica" is excerpted from "Necrobiosis Lipoidica," Genetic and Rare Diseases Information Center (GARD), National Center for Advancing Translational Sciences (NCATS), June 6, 2016.

hyperinsulinemia through diet and medication, losing weight with obesity-associated AN, removing or treating a tumor, or stopping medications that cause AN.

Prevalence of Acanthosis Nigricans

Due to the rising prevalence of obesity and diabetes a high prevalence of acanthosis nigricans (AN) has been observed recently. The prevalence varies from 7 to 74 percent, according to age, race, frequency of type, degree of obesity, and concomitant endocrinopathy. It is most common in Native Americans, followed by African Americans, Hispanics, and Caucasians. Malignant AN is less common.

(Source: "An Approach to Acanthosis Nigricans," National Center for Biotechnology Information (NCBI).)

Necrobiosis Lipoidica

Necrobiosis lipoidica is a rare skin disorder of collagen degeneration. It is characterized by a rash that occurs on the lower legs. It is more common in women, and there are usually several spots. They are slightly raised shiny red-brown patches. The centers are often yellowish and may develop open sores that are slow to heal. Infections can occur but are uncommon. Some patients have itching, pain, or abnormal sensations. It usually occurs more often in people with diabetes and in people with a family history of diabetes or a tendency to get diabetes, but it can occur in nondiabetic people. About 11 to 65 percent of patients with necrobiosis lipoidica also have diabetes, but the exact cause is still not known. Treatment is difficult. The disease is typically chronic with variable progression and scarring.

Incidence Rates of Necrobiosis Lipoidica

Incidence rates are higher in women than men and in adults than children. Necrobiosis lipoidica typically presents at 30 to 40 years of age. It appears to be a discernible association between necrobiosis lipoidica (NL) and diabetes mellitus in numerous studies; however, diabetic patients also suffering from NL are less than one percent. Two other studies, on the other hand, regard 80 and 60 percent of NL patients to be diabetic, respectively.

(Source: "Treatment Modalities of Necrobiosis Lipoidica: A Concise Systematic Review," National Center for Biotechnology Information (NCBI).)

Chapter 32

Sexual and Bladder Problems of Diabetes

Sexual problems and bladder problems are common as people age, but diabetes can make these problems worse. You or your partner may have trouble having or enjoying sex. Or, you may leak urine or have trouble emptying your bladder normally.

Blood vessels and nerves can be damaged by the effects of high blood glucose, also called "blood sugar." This damage can lead to sexual and bladder problems. Keeping your blood glucose levels in your target range is an important way to prevent damage to your blood vessels and nerves.

Work with your healthcare team to help prevent or treat sexual and bladder problems. These problems may be signs that you need to manage your diabetes in a different way. Remember, a healthy sex life and a healthy bladder can improve your quality of life, so take action now if you have concerns.

Can Sexual and Bladder Problems Be Symptoms of Diabetes?

Yes. Changes in sexual function or bladder habits may be a sign that you have diabetes. Nerve damage caused by diabetes, also called "diabetic neuropathy," can damage parts of your body—such as your genitals or urinary tract. For example, men with diabetes may develop erectile dysfunction (ED) 10 to 15 years earlier than men without diabetes.

About This Chapter: This chapter includes text excerpted from "Diabetes, Sexual, and Bladder Problems," National Institute of Diabetes and Digestive and Kidney Diseases (NIDDK), June 2018.

Talk with a healthcare professional if you have any symptoms of diabetes, including sexual and bladder problems.

When Should I See a Doctor about My Sexual or Bladder Problems?

See a healthcare professional for problems with sex or your bladder. These problems could be a sign that you need to manage your diabetes differently. You may find it embarrassing and difficult to talk about these things. However, remember that healthcare professionals are trained to speak with people about every kind of health problem. Everyone deserves to have healthy relationships and enjoy the activities they love.

What Makes Me More Likely to Develop Sexual or Bladder Problems?

You are more likely to develop sexual or bladder problems if you have diabetes and:

- Have high blood glucose that is not well controlled, also called "high blood sugar"
- Have nerve damage
- Have high blood pressure that is not treated
- Have high cholesterol that is not treated
- Are overweight or have obesity
- Are not physically active
- Are taking certain medicines
- Drink too many alcoholic drinks
- Smoke

Research also suggests that certain genes may make people more likely to develop diabetic neuropathy.

What Sexual Problems Can Men with Diabetes Have?

Changes in your blood vessels, nerves, hormones, and emotional health during diabetes may make it more difficult for you to have satisfactory sex. Diabetes and its related challenges also may make it harder for you to have a child.

Erectile Dysfunction

You have ED if you are unable to get or keep an erection firm enough for satisfactory sexual intercourse. More than half of men with diabetes will get ED. Men who have diabetes are more than three times more likely to develop ED than men who do not have diabetes. Good diabetes management may help prevent and treat ED caused by nerve damage and circulation problems. A doctor can help treat ED with medicine or a change in your diabetes care plan.

Retrograde Ejaculation

Rarely, diabetes can cause retrograde ejaculation, which is when part or all of your semen goes into your bladder instead of out of your penis during ejaculation. During retrograde ejaculation, semen enters your bladder, mixes with urine, and is safely urinated out. A urine sample after ejaculation can show if you have retrograde ejaculation. Some men with retrograde ejaculation may not ejaculate at all.

Penile Curvature

Men with diabetes are more likely to have Peyronie disease, also called "penile curvature," than men who do not have diabetes. Men with Peyronie disease have scar tissue, called a "plaque," in the penis, making it curve when erect. Curves in the penis can make sexual intercourse painful or difficult. Some men with Peyronie disease may have ED.

Low Testosterone

Men's testosterone levels naturally lower with age. However, lower-than-normal testosterone levels may be the cause of some men's ED or can explain why some men often feel tired, depressed, or have a low sex drive. Men with diabetes, especially those who are older and overweight, are more likely to have low testosterone, or "low T."

If your doctor thinks you might have low T, you will probably be asked to give a blood sample, and a healthcare professional will give you a physical exam. Your doctor may suggest treating your low testosterone with a prescription gel, injection, or patch.

Several studies show that, along with good diabetes management, testosterone therapy can lessen a man's sexual problems. However, testosterone therapy may have serious risks and may not be safe for all men. Talk with your doctor about testosterone therapy side effects and whether it is right for you.

Fertility Problems

Some studies show that men with diabetes can have problems with their sperm that make it harder to conceive. Your sperm could be slow or not move well, or your sperm may not be able to fertilize a woman's egg well. Working closely with your partner and a healthcare professional trained in fertility issues may help.

If you and your partner want to conceive a child, your doctor may treat retrograde ejaculation caused by diabetes with medicine or by changing your diabetes care plan. Or, talk with a urologist who is a fertility expert. She or he may be able to collect your sperm from your urine and then use it for artificial insemination.

What Sexual Problems Can Women with Diabetes Have?

Low sexual desire and response, vaginal dryness, and painful sex can be caused by nerve damage, reduced blood flow to the genitals, and hormonal changes. Other conditions can cause these problems too, including menopause. If you notice a change in your sex life, talk with your healthcare team. A physical exam, which will include a pelvic exam and blood and urine tests, may help your doctor find the cause of your problems.

Low Sexual Desire and Response

Low sexual desire and sexual response can include:

- Being unable to become or stay aroused

- Not having enough vaginal lubrication

- Having little to no feeling in your genitals

- Being unable to have an orgasm or rarely having one

With diabetes, your body and mind will likely go through many changes. For example, both high and low blood glucose levels can affect how and if you become aroused. Or, you may find yourself more tired than usual or depressed and anxious, making you less interested in sex.

Your healthcare team can help you make changes to your diabetes care plan so that you are back on track. Women who keep blood glucose levels in their target range are less likely to have nerve damage, which can lead to low sexual desire and response.

Painful Sex

Some women with diabetes say that they have uncomfortable or painful sexual intercourse. The nerves that tell your vagina to lubricate during stimulation can become damaged by diabetes. A prescription or over-the-counter (OTC) vaginal lubricant may help if you have vaginal dryness. Managing your blood glucose well over many weeks, months, and years can help prevent nerve damage.

Yeast and Bladder Infections

Women with diabetes are more likely to have yeast infections because yeast organisms can grow more easily when your blood glucose levels are higher. Yeast infections can be uncomfortable or painful and prevent you from enjoying activities, including having sex.

Although some yeast infections can be treated at home, talk with a healthcare professional first about your symptoms. Some symptoms of yeast infections are similar to other types of infections, including sexually transmitted diseases (STDs).

Pregnancy Concerns and Fertility Problems

If you have diabetes and plan to become pregnant, it is important to get your blood glucose levels close to your target range before you get pregnant. High blood glucose can harm a fetus during the first weeks of pregnancy, even before you know you are pregnant.

If you have diabetes and are already pregnant, see your doctor as soon as possible to make a plan to manage your diabetes. Working with your healthcare team and following your diabetes management plan can help you have a healthy pregnancy and a healthy baby.

Conditions such as obesity and polycystic ovarian syndrome (PCOS) that are linked to diabetes can make it harder to conceive a child. Talk with a healthcare professional, such as a gynecologist or a fertility specialist, if you are having problems conceiving a child.

What Bladder Problems Can Men and Women with Diabetes Have?

Diabetes can cause nerve damage to your urinary tract, causing bladder problems. Overweight and obesity also can increase bladder problems, such as urinary incontinence (UI). Managing diabetes is an important part of preventing problems that can lead to excess urination.

Your healthcare team may be able to help you manage your blood glucose levels and help you lose weight if needed. Doctors use blood and urine tests to diagnose bladder problems or conditions with similar symptoms. Doctors also may use urodynamic testing to see what kind of bladder problem you have.

Frequent and Urgent Urination

Some people with diabetes who regularly have high blood glucose levels may have to urinate too often, also called "urinary frequency." Even men and women with diabetes who manage their blood glucose levels within their target range sometimes feel the sudden urge to urinate, called "urgency incontinence." This can happen at night also. Medicines may help reduce the symptoms of bladder control problems.

Trouble "Going"

You may find that diabetes causes you to no longer feel when your bladder is full. Many people with diabetes report that they have trouble "going." Over time, having a too-full bladder can cause damage to your bladder muscles that push urine out. When these muscles do not work correctly, urine may stay in your bladder too long, also called "urinary retention." Urinary retention can cause bladder infections, urine leaks, and the feeling that you always have to go.

Leaking Urine

People with diabetes are more likely to have other types of UI, such as stress incontinence. Nerve damage, obesity, and bladder infections, which are linked with diabetes, are often related to bladder control problems. Leaking urine can cause you to avoid activities you once enjoyed, including sex.

If you are overweight, losing weight can help you have fewer leaks. Avoiding weight gain may prevent UI. Studies suggest that, as your body mass index (BMI) increases, you are more likely to leak. If you are overweight or have obesity, talk with your doctor about how to lose weight.

Work with your healthcare team to help manage and prevent urine leaks. Bladder control problems are often treatable and are very common, even in people who do not have diabetes. You do not have to accept rushing to the bathroom all the time to avoid leaks.

Bladder Infections

People with diabetes are more likely to have urinary tract infections, also called "bladder infections," or "cystitis." See a doctor right away if you have frequent, urgent urination that may be painful. Bladder infections can develop into kidney infections and can make bladder symptoms, such as leaks and urine retention, worse. Also, bladder infections can get in the way of your everyday life, including intimacy. Managing your blood glucose levels can help prevent bladder infections.

How Can I Prevent and Treat My Sexual or Bladder Problems?

Managing your diabetes can help prevent nerve damage and other diabetes problems that can lead to sexual and bladder problems. With your healthcare team, you can help prevent and treat your sexual or bladder control problems by:

- Keeping your blood glucose, blood pressure, and cholesterol levels close to your target numbers

- Being physically active

- Keeping a healthy weight

- Quitting smoking if you smoke

- Getting help for any emotional or psychological problems

Sex is a physical activity, so be sure to check your blood glucose level before and after sex, especially if you take insulin. Both high blood glucose levels and low blood glucose levels can cause problems during sex.

Counseling may also be helpful when you notice changes in your sexual function or desire. These types of changes are very common as people age or adjust to health problems.

If you have a partner, she or he also may be an important member of your healthcare team. You may find it helpful to share your concerns and have that person join you at the doctor's office or at counseling. Your friends and family may also be able to support you if you are having bladder problems.

Part Four
Mental Health and Lifestyle Issues

Chapter 33

The Link between Diabetes and Mental Health

Mental health affects so many aspects of daily life—how you think and feel, handle stress, relate to others, and make choices. You can see how having a mental-health problem could make it harder to stick to your diabetes care plan.

The Mind–Body Connection

Thoughts, feelings, beliefs, and attitudes can affect how healthy your body is. Untreated mental-health issues can make diabetes worse, and problems with diabetes can make mental-health issues worse. But, fortunately if one gets better, the other tends to get better too.

Depression: More than Just a Bad Mood

Depression is a medical illness that causes feelings of sadness and often a loss of interest in activities you used to enjoy. It can get in the way of how well you function at work and home, including taking care of your diabetes. When you are not able to manage your diabetes well, your risk goes up for diabetes complications, such as heart disease and nerve damage.

People with diabetes are 2 to 3 times more likely to have depression than people without diabetes. Only 25 to 50 percent of people with diabetes who have depression get diagnosed and treated. But, treatment—therapy, medicine, or both—is usually very effective. And without treatment, depression often gets worse, not better.

About This Chapter: This chapter includes text excerpted from "Diabetes and Mental Health," Centers for Disease Control and Prevention (CDC), August 6, 2018.

Symptoms of depression can be mild to severe, and include:

- Feeling sad or empty

- Losing interest in favorite activities

- Overeating or not wanting to eat at all

- Not being able to sleep or sleeping too much

- Having trouble concentrating or making decisions

- Feeling very tired

- Feeling hopeless, irritable, anxious, or guilty

- Having aches or pains, headaches, cramps, or digestive problems

- Having thoughts of suicide or death

If you think you might have depression, get in touch with your doctor right away for help getting treatment. The earlier depression is treated, the better for you, your quality of life, and your diabetes.

Questions to ask your doctor if you think you may be depressed:

- I'm worried that I may be depressed. What can I do to feel better?
- What can I expect if you send me to talk with a mental health professional?
- What kind of medicine helps with depression?
- If I am given medicine for depression, how long will it take for me to feel better?

(Source: "Living a Balanced Life with Diabetes: Depression Checklist," Centers for Disease Control and Prevention (CDC).)

Stress and Anxiety

Stress is part of life, from traffic jams to family demands to everyday diabetes care. You can feel stress as an emotion, such as fear or anger; as a physical reaction, such as sweating or a racing heart; or both.

If you are stressed, you may not take as good care of yourself as usual. Your blood sugar levels can be affected too—stress hormones make blood sugar rise or fall unpredictably, and stress from being sick or injured can make your blood sugar go up. Being stressed for a long time can lead to other health problems or make them worse.

Anxiety—feelings of worry, fear, or being on edge—is how your mind and body react to stress. People with diabetes are 20 percent more likely than those without diabetes to have anxiety at some point in their life. Managing a long-term condition like diabetes is a major source of anxiety for some.

Studies show that therapy for anxiety usually works better than medicine, but sometimes both together works best. You can also help lower your stress and anxiety by:

- Getting active. Even a quick walk can be calming, and the effect can last for hours.

- Doing some relaxation exercises, such as meditation or yoga

- Calling or texting a friend who understands you (not someone who is causing you stress).

- Grabbing some "you" time. Take a break from whatever you are doing. Go outside, read something fun—whatever helps you recharge.

- Limiting alcohol and caffeine, eating healthy food, and getting enough sleep.

Anxiety can feel like low blood sugar and vice versa. It may be hard for you to recognize which it is and treat it effectively. If you are feeling anxious, try checking your blood sugar and treat it if it is low.

There will always be some stress in life. But, if you feel overwhelmed, talking to a mental-health counselor can help. Ask your doctor for a referral.

Diabetes Distress

You may sometimes feel discouraged, worried, frustrated, or tired of dealing with daily diabetes care; it is like diabetes is controlling you instead of the other way around. Maybe you have been trying hard but not seeing results. Or you have developed a health problem related to diabetes in spite of your best efforts.

Those overwhelming feelings, known as "diabetes distress," may cause you to slip into unhealthy habits, stop checking your blood sugar, or even skip doctor's appointments. It happens to many—if not most—people with diabetes, often after years of good management. In any 18-month period, 33 to 50 percent of people with diabetes have diabetes distress.

Diabetes distress can look like depression or anxiety, but it cannot be treated effectively with medicine. Instead, these approaches have been shown to help:

- Make sure you are seeing an endocrinologist for your diabetes care. She or he is likely to have a deeper understanding of diabetes challenges than your regular doctor.

- Ask your doctor to refer you to a mental-health counselor who specializes in chronic health conditions.

- Get some one-on-one time with a diabetes educator so you can problem-solve together.

- Focus on one or two small diabetes management goals instead of thinking you have to work on everything all at once.

- Join a diabetes support group so you can share your thoughts and feelings with people who have the same concerns (and learn from them too).

Chapter 34

Tips for Coping with Diabetes Distress

Managing diabetes can be hard. Sometimes you may feel overwhelmed. Having diabetes means that you need to check your blood sugar levels often, make healthy food choices, be physically active, remember to take your medicine, and make other good decisions about your health several times a day. In addition, you may also worry about having low or high blood sugar levels; the costs of your medicines; and developing diabetes-related complications, such as heart disease or nerve damage.

When all of this feels like too much to deal with, you may have something called "diabetes distress." This is when all the worry, frustration, anger, and burnout makes it hard for you to take care of yourself and keep up with the daily demands of diabetes.

The good news is that there are things you can do to cope with diabetes and manage stress. Here are 10 tips that can help.

1. **Pay attention to your feelings.** Almost everyone feels frustrated or stressed from time to time. Dealing with diabetes can add to these feelings and make you feel overwhelmed. Having these feelings for more than a week or two may signal that you need help coping with your diabetes so that you can feel better.

2. **Talk with your healthcare providers about your feelings.** Let your doctor, nurse, diabetes educator, psychologist, or social worker know how you have been feeling. They can help you problem-solve your concerns about diabetes. They may also suggest that you speak with other healthcare providers to get help.

About This Chapter: This chapter includes text excerpted from "10 Tips for Coping with Diabetes Distress," Centers for Disease Control and Prevention (CDC), December 6, 2017.

3. **Talk to your healthcare providers about negative reactions other people may have about your diabetes.** Your healthcare providers can help you manage feelings of being judged by others because you have diabetes. It is important not to feel that you have to hide your diabetes from other people.

4. **Ask if help is available for the costs of diabetes medicines and supplies.** If you are worried about the cost of your medicines, talk with your pharmacist and other health-care providers. They may know about government or other programs that can assist people with costs. You can also check with community health centers to see if they know about programs that help people get insulin, diabetes medicines, and supplies (test strips, syringes, etc.).

5. **Talk with your family and friends.** Tell those closest to you how you feel about having diabetes. Be honest about the problems you are having in dealing with diabetes. Just telling others how you feel helps to relieve some of the stress. However, some-times, the people around you may add to your stress. Let them know how and when you need them to help you.

6. **Allow loved ones to help you take care of your diabetes.** Those closest to you can help you in several ways. They can remind you to take your medicines, help monitor your blood sugar levels, join you in being physically active, and prepare healthy meals. They can also learn about diabetes and go with you when you visit your doctor. Ask your loved ones to help with your diabetes in ways that are useful to you.

7. **Talk to other people with diabetes.** Other people with diabetes understand some of the things you are going through. Ask them how they deal with their diabe-tes and what works for them. They can help you feel less lonely and overwhelmed. Ask your healthcare providers about diabetes support groups in your community or online.

8. **Do one thing at a time.** When you think about everything you need to do to manage your diabetes, it can be overwhelming. To deal with diabetes distress, make a list of all of the tasks you have to do to take care of yourself each day. Try to work on each task separately, one at a time.

9. **Pace yourself.** As you work on your goals, such as increasing physical activity, take it slowly. You do not have to meet your goals immediately. Your goal may be to walk 10 minutes 3 times a day each day of the week, but you can start by walking 2 times a day or every other day.

10. **Take time to do things you enjoy.** Give yourself a break. Set aside time in your day to do something you really love; it could be calling a friend, playing a game, or working on a fun project. Find out about activities near you that you can do with a friend.

Remember that it is important to pay attention to your feelings. If you notice that you are feeling frustrated, tired, and unable to make decisions about your diabetes care, take action. Tell your family, friends, and healthcare providers. They can help you get the support you need.

Chapter 35

Diabetes Management at School

Maintaining Optimal Blood Glucose Control

The goal of effective diabetes management is to keep blood glucose levels within a target range determined by the student's personal diabetes healthcare team. Optimal blood glucose control helps to promote normal growth and development and to prevent the immediate dangers of blood glucose levels that are too high or too low. Maintaining blood glucose levels within the target range also can help to optimize the student's ability to learn by avoiding the effects of hypoglycemia (low blood glucose level) and hyperglycemia (high blood glucose level) on cognition, attention, and behavior. In the long term, effective diabetes management helps to prevent or delay the serious complications of diabetes, such as heart disease, stroke, blindness, kidney failure, gum disease, nerve disease, and amputations of the foot or leg.

The key to maintaining optimal blood glucose control is to carefully balance food intake, physical activity, insulin, and/or other medication. As a general rule, food makes blood glucose levels go up. Physical activity, insulin, and diabetes medications make blood glucose levels go down. Several other factors, such as growth and puberty, physical and emotional stress, illness, or injury, also can affect blood glucose levels.

Many students with diabetes check their blood glucose levels throughout the day using a blood glucose meter. Some students also wear a continuous glucose monitor (CGM). When blood glucose levels are too low or too high, corrective actions need to be taken.

About This Chapter: This chapter includes text excerpted from "What Is Effective Diabetes Management at School?" National Institute of Diabetes and Digestive and Kidney Diseases (NIDDK), November 1, 2016.

Assisting the Student with Performing Diabetes Care Tasks

Diabetes management is needed 24 hours a day, 7 days a week. Many students will be able to handle all or almost all of their nonemergency diabetes care tasks by themselves. Others, because of age, developmental level, inexperience, or issues with adherence to their diabetes tasks, will need help from school personnel.

All students with diabetes will need help during an emergency, which may happen at any time. School personnel need to be prepared to provide diabetes care at school and at all school-sponsored activities in which a student with diabetes participates.

The school nurse is the most appropriate person in the school setting to provide care for a student with diabetes. Many schools, however, do not have a full-time nurse, and sometimes a single nurse must cover more than one school. Moreover, even when a nurse is assigned to a school full time, she or he may not always be available during the school day, during extracurricular activities, or on field trips. In circumstances where a nurse is absent or unavailable, the school remains responsible for arranging and implementing the agreed upon diabetes care that is necessary to enable the child to participate in school and school-related activities. The school nurse or another qualified healthcare professional plays a major role in selecting and training appropriate staff and providing professional supervision and consultation regarding routine and emergency care of the student with diabetes.

Backpack Checklist

Create a backpack checklist that the student can use every day to be sure all necessary supplies are packed:

- Blood sugar meter and extra batteries, testing strips, lancets
- Ketone testing supplies
- Insulin and syringes/pens (include for backup even if an insulin pump is used)
- Antiseptic wipes
- Water
- Glucose tablets or other fast-acting carbs like fruit juice or hard candy (about 10 to 15 grams) that will raise blood sugar levels quickly

(Source: "Managing Diabetes at School," Centers for Disease Control and Prevention (CDC).)

Designating Trained Diabetes Personnel

Nonmedical school personnel—called "trained diabetes personnel" in this chapter—can be trained and supervised to perform diabetes care tasks safely in the school setting. School staff who may be trained to provide diabetes care include: health aides, teachers, physical education personnel, school principals, school secretaries, school psychologists or guidance counselors, food service personnel, and other appropriate personnel. Some schools may call these individuals "unlicensed assistive personnel," "assistive personnel," "paraprofessionals," or "trained nonmedical personnel." Trained diabetes personnel may be identified from existing school staff who are willing to serve in this role.

Care tasks performed by trained diabetes personnel may include blood glucose monitoring, insulin administration (by syringe, pen, or assistance with a pump), glucagon administration, ketone testing, and basic carbohydrate counting. In addition to learning how to perform general diabetes care tasks, trained diabetes personnel should receive student-specific training, and they should be supervised by the school nurse or another qualified healthcare professional.

The school nurse has a critical role in training and supervising trained diabetes personnel to ensure the health and safety of students with diabetes. In addition, a student's healthcare provider or a diabetes educator may assist in training nonmedical personnel in diabetes care. Given the rapid changes in diabetes technology, therapies, and evidence-based practice, the school nurse who provides care to students with diabetes and facilitates diabetes management training for school personnel has the professional responsibility to acquire and maintain knowledge and competency related to diabetes management.

Once it has been determined that a student-specific diabetes care task may be delegated, the school nurse should be involved in the decision-making process to identify which school personnel are most appropriate to be trained. A diabetes-trained healthcare professional, such as a school nurse or a certified diabetes educator, develops and implements the training program, evaluates the ability of the trained diabetes personnel to perform the task, and establishes a plan for ongoing supervision throughout the school year. Diabetes care must be carried out as specified in the student's healthcare plans.

Chapter 36

Importance of Wearing Medical Alert Bracelets and Necklaces

Medical alert bracelets and necklaces, also known as "personal identification jewelry," are tags that people with certain illness, including diabetes, wear to save their lives in case of a medical emergency. The bracelets or necklaces are engraved with critical information such as the patient's personal details and medical conditions.

How the Medical Alert Bracelet Works

Patients with diabetes may sometimes face adverse conditions such as a sudden drop in blood glucose level, dizziness, and loss of consciousness, during which time the patients may not be able to express themselves clearly and seek medical help. In such situations, medical alert jewelry will be helpful in conveying the message that the wearer is suffering from a specific illness and may need immediate medical aid.

Information to Put on a Medical Alert Bracelet

Medical information such as the person's medical condition ("diabetes"), allergies to any food or medicine, and life-saving medicines should be engraved boldly on one side of the jewelry for easy identification. The other side should contain other necessary information, such as:

- Patient's name
- Blood type

About This Chapter: "Importance of Wearing Medical Alert Bracelets and Necklaces," © 2018 Omnigraphics. Reviewed June 2019.

- Name of physician

- Emergency contact information, and so on.

Information provided on the jewelry should be simple and precise and abbreviations of medical terms should be used to save room. When using abbreviations, however, make sure that they comply with international medical standards. Also, pay attention to the use of upper- and lower-case letters of the alphabet in the abbreviations.

Diabetes Goes Digital

Keeping track of food, fitness, blood sugar levels … it's a lot to manage. But there's help—for free—right at your fingertips. A quick online search will turn up hundreds of apps and websites that make it easier to:

- Track blood sugar and share results with your family, friends, and healthcare team.

- Meet other people with diabetes through online forums and community groups.

- Access tried-and-true calorie and carb tracking software to support healthy, sustainable weight loss.

- Help kids with type 1 diabetes learn about healthy eating using interactive games and other activities.

(Source: "Diabetes Goes Digital," Centers for Disease Control and Prevention (CDC).)

Benefits of Medical Alert Jewelry

- Acts as a tool to convey the medical condition of the patient in case of emergencies

- Ensures quick recognition of ailments, allergies, and medications, and facilitates prompt diagnosis

- Ensures appropriate and timely medical care

- Reduces potentially harmful medical errors at the time of admission and discharge

How to Buy a Medical Alert Jewelry

Medical alert jewelry is available in most of surgical supply stores and many pharmacies. It is also available online on many websites. The jewelry is usually made of metals such as gold, silver, or stainless steel. However, nonmetallic jewelry made of leather, rubber, or nylon is also available. These nonmetallic bracelets are more popular among youth and are suitable for those who have skin sensitivity to metals. Although the bracelets come in different colors and designs, it is always preferable to choose the simpler ones because the simpler the design, the easier it is to read the message contained on it.

References

1. "The Basics of Medical Alert Bracelets," StickyJ Medical ID, October 25, 2017.

2. "Importance of Medical IDs," MedicAlert Foundation, October 10, 2014.

3. "The Benefits of Wearing a Medical ID Bracelet," MyIDShop, September 21, 2017.

4. "Importance of Wearing a Medical Alert Bracelet with Diabetes," Joslin Diabetes Center, October 17, 2008.

Chapter 37

Driving When You Have Diabetes

For most people, driving represents freedom, control, and competence. Driving enables most people to get to the places they want or need to go. For many people, driving is important economically—some drive as part of their job or to get to and from work.

Driving is a complex skill. Our ability to drive safely can be affected by changes in our physical, emotional, and mental condition.

How Can Having Diabetes Affect My Driving?

- In the short term, diabetes can make your blood glucose (sugar) levels too high or too low. As a result, diabetes can make you:

  - Feel sleepy or dizzy

  - Feel confused

  - Have blurred vision

  - Lose consciousness or have a seizure

- In the long run, diabetes can lead to problems that affect driving. Diabetes may cause nerve damage in your hands, legs, and feet, or eyes. In some cases, diabetes can cause blindness or lead to amputation.

About This Chapter: This chapter includes text excerpted from "Driving When You Have Diabetes," National Highway Traffic Safety Administration (NHTSA), November 15, 2003. Reviewed June 2019.

Can I Still Drive with Diabetes?

Yes, people with diabetes are able to drive unless they are limited by certain complications of diabetes. These include severely low blood glucose levels or vision problems. If you are experiencing diabetes-related complications, you should work closely with your diabetes healthcare team to find out if diabetes affects your ability to drive. If it does, discuss if there are actions you can take to continue to drive safely.

What Can I Do to Ensure That I Can Drive Safely with Diabetes?

- Insulin and some oral medications can cause blood glucose levels to become dangerously low (hypoglycemia). Do not drive if your blood glucose level is too low. If you do, you might not be able to make good choices, focus on your driving, or control your car. Your healthcare team can help you determine when you should check your blood glucose level before driving and how often you should check while driving.

- Make sure you always carry your blood glucose meter and plenty of snacks (including a quick-acting source of glucose) with you. Pull over as soon as you feel any of the signs of a low blood glucose level. Check your blood glucose.

- If your glucose level is low, eat a snack that contains a fast-acting sugar, such as juice, soda with sugar (not diet), hard candy, or glucose tablets. Wait 15 minutes, and then check your blood glucose again. Treat again as needed. Once your glucose level has risen to your target range, eat a more substantial snack or meal containing protein. Do not continue driving until your blood glucose level has improved.

- Most people with diabetes experience warning signs of a low blood glucose level. However, if you experience hypoglycemia without advance warning, you should not drive. Talk to your healthcare team about how glycemic awareness training might help you sense the beginning stages of hypoglycemia.

- In extreme situations, high blood glucose levels (hyperglycemia) also may affect driving. Talk to your healthcare team if you have a history of very high glucose levels to determine at what point such levels might affect your ability to be a safe driver.

- The key to preventing diabetes-related eye problems is a good control of blood glucose levels, good blood pressure control, and good eye care. A yearly exam with an eye care professional is essential.

- If you are experiencing long-term complications of diabetes, such as vision or sensation problems, or if you have had an amputation, your diabetes healthcare team can refer you to a driving specialist. This specialist can give you on and off-road tests to see if, and how, your diabetes is affecting your driving. The specialist also may offer training to improve your driving skills.

- Improving your driving skills could help keep you and others around you safe. To find a specialist near you, call the Association of Driver Rehabilitation Specialists (ADED) at 800-290-2344 or go to their website at www.aded.net. You also can call hospitals and rehabilitation facilities to find an occupational therapist who can help with the driving skills assessment.

What If I Have to Cut Back or Give Up Driving?

- You can keep your independence even if you have to cut back or give up on your driving. It may take planning ahead on your part, but planning will help get you to the places you need to go and to the people you want to see.

- Consider:
  - Rides with family and friends
  - Taxi cabs
  - Shuttle buses or vans
  - Public buses, trains, and subways
  - Walking

Where Do I Find Out More about Diabetes?

Your first step is to talk with your diabetes healthcare team. You also can contact the:

American Diabetes Association (ADA)
800-342-2383
www.diabetes.org

National Diabetes Information Clearinghouse (NDIC)
800-860-8747
www.diabetes.niddk.nih.gov

Healthfinder
www.healthfinder.gov

Wear Your Safety Belt

Always wear your safety belt when you are driving or riding in a car. Make sure that every person who is riding with you also is buckled up. Wear your safety belt even if your car has airbags.

Chapter 38

Traveling When You Have Diabetes

Traveling to new places gets you out of your routine—that is a big part of the fun. But, delayed meals, unfamiliar food, being more active than usual, and different time zones can all disrupt diabetes management. Plan ahead so you can count on more fun and less worry on the way and when you get to your destination.

Before You Go

- Visit your doctor for a checkup to ensure that you are fit for the trip. Make sure to ask your doctor:

    - How your planned activities could affect your diabetes and what to do about it

    - How to adjust your insulin doses if you are traveling to a different time zone

    - To provide prescriptions for your medicines in case you lose them or run out

    - If you will need any vaccines

    - To write a letter stating that you have diabetes and why you need your medical supplies

- Just in case, locate pharmacies and clinics close to where you are staying.

- Get a medical ID bracelet that states you have diabetes and any other health conditions.

- Get travel insurance in case you miss your flight or need medical care.

- Order a special meal for the flight that fits with your meal plan, or pack your own.

About This Chapter: This chapter includes text excerpted from "21 Tips for Traveling with Diabetes," Centers for Disease Control and Prevention (CDC), September 17, 2018.

- Packing:

  - Put your diabetes supplies in a carry-on bag (insulin could get too cold in your checked luggage). Think about bringing a smaller bag to have at your seat for insulin, glucose tablets, and snacks.

  - Pack twice as much medicine as you think you will need. Carry medicines in the pharmacy bottles they came in, or ask your pharmacist to print out extra labels you can attach to plastic bags.

  - Be sure to pack healthy snacks, such as fruit, raw veggies, and nuts.

- Airport security:

  - Get an optional Transportation Security Administration (TSA) to help the screening process go more quickly and smoothly.

  - Good news: People with diabetes are exempt from the 3.4 oz. the liquid rule for medicines; fast-acting carbs, such as juice; and gel packs to keep insulin cool.

  - A continuous glucose monitor or insulin pump could be damaged going through the X-ray machine*. You do not have to disconnect from either; ask for a hand inspection instead.

A machine that uses high-energy radiation to diagnose diseases by making pictures of the inside of the body.

Do not leave home without these items:
- Doctor's letter and prescriptions
- Snacks and glucose tablets
- Extra insulin and diabetes medicines

While You Are Traveling

- If you are driving, pack a cooler with healthy foods and plenty of water to drink.

- Do not store insulin or diabetes medicine in direct sunlight or in a hot car; keep them in the cooler too. Do not put insulin directly on ice or a gel pack.

- Heat can also damage your blood sugar monitor, insulin pump, and other diabetes equipment. Do not leave them in a hot car, by a pool, in direct sunlight, or on the beach. The same goes for supplies such as test strips.

- You can find healthy food options at the airport or a roadside restaurant:

  - Fruit, nuts, sandwiches, yogurt

  - Salads with chicken or fish (skip the dried fruit and croutons)

  - Eggs and omelets

  - Burgers with a lettuce wrap instead of a bun

  - Fajitas (skip the tortillas and rice)

- Stop and get out of the car, or walk up and down the aisle of the plane or train every hour or two to prevent blood clots (people with diabetes are at a higher risk).

- Set an alarm on your phone for taking medicine if you are traveling across time zones.

Once You Are There

- Your blood sugar may be out of your target range at first, but your body should adjust in a few days. Check your blood sugar often, and treat highs or lows as instructed by your doctor or diabetes educator.

- If you are going to be more active than usual, check your blood sugar before and after, and make adjustments to food, activity, and insulin as needed.

- Food is a huge highlight (and temptation) on a cruise. Avoid the giant buffet, and instead, order off the spa menu (healthier choices) or low-carb menu (most ships have one), or order something tasty that fits in your meal plan from the 24-hour room service.

- Do not overdo physical activity during the heat of the day. Avoid getting a sunburn, and do not go barefoot, not even on the beach.

- High temperatures can change how your body uses insulin. You may need to test your blood sugar more often and adjust your insulin dose and what you eat and drink.

- You may not be able to find everything you need to manage your diabetes away from home, especially in another country. Learn some useful phrases, such as "I have diabetes" and "where is the nearest pharmacy?"

- If your vacation is in the great outdoors, bring wet wipes so you can clean your hands before you check your blood sugar.

Chapter 39

Take Care of Your Diabetes during Sick Days and Special Times

Diabetes is part of your life. You can learn how to take care of yourself and your diabetes when you are sick, when you are at school or work, when you are away from home, when an emergency or a natural disaster happens, or when you are thinking about having a baby or are pregnant.

When You Are Sick

Having a cold, the flu, or an infection can raise your blood glucose levels. Being sick puts stress on your body. Your body releases hormones to deal with the stress and to fight the sickness. Higher hormone levels can also cause high blood glucose levels. You should have a plan for managing your diabetes when you are sick. The first step is to talk with your healthcare team and write down:

- How often to check your blood glucose levels

- Whether you should check for ketones in your blood or urine

- Whether you should change the usual dose of your diabetes medicines

- What to eat and drink

- When to call your doctor

About This Chapter: This chapter includes text excerpted from "Take Care of Your Diabetes during Sick Days and Special Times," National Institute of Diabetes and Digestive and Kidney Diseases (NIDDK), February 2014. Reviewed June 2019.

People who are sick sometimes feel as though they cannot eat as much or cannot keep food down, which can cause low blood glucose levels. Consuming carbohydrate-rich drinks or snacks can help prevent low blood glucose.

If you are sick, your healthcare team may recommend the following:

- Check your blood glucose levels at least four times a day, and write down the results in your record book. Keep your results handy so you can report the results to your healthcare team.

- Keep taking your diabetes medicines, even if you cannot eat.

- Drink at least 1 cup, or 8 ounces, of water or other calorie-free, caffeine-free liquid every hour while you are awake.

- If you cannot eat your usual food, try eating or drinking any of the following to prevent low blood glucose levels:

  - Juice

  - Saltine crackers

  - Dry toast

  - Soup

  - Broth or bouillon

  - Ice pops or sherbet

  - Gelatin that is not sugar-free

  - Milk

  - Yogurt

  - Soda that is not sugar-free

Your doctor may ask that you call right away if:

- Your blood glucose levels are above 240 even though you have taken your diabetes medicines.

- Your urine or blood ketone levels are above normal.

- You vomit more than once.

- You have diarrhea for more than six hours.

- You have trouble breathing.

- You have a high fever.

- You cannot think clearly or you feel more drowsy than usual.

- You should call your doctor if you have questions about taking care of yourself.

Action Steps If You Take Insulin

- Take your insulin, even if you are sick and have been throwing up.
- Ask your healthcare team about how to adjust your insulin dose based on your blood glucose test results.

Action Steps If You Do not Take Insulin

- Take your diabetes medicines, even if you are sick and have been throwing up.

When You Are at School or Work

Take care of your diabetes when you are at school or at work:

- Follow your healthy eating plan.

- Take your medicines, and check your blood glucose levels as usual.

- Tell your teachers, friends, or close coworkers that you have diabetes and teach them about the signs of low blood glucose. You may need their help if your blood glucose levels drop too low.

- Keep snacks nearby and carry some with you at all times to treat low blood glucose.

- If you have trained diabetes staff at your school or work, tell them that you have diabetes.

- Wear or carry an identification tag or card that says you have diabetes.

When You Are Away from Home

These tips can help you when you are away from home:

- Get all your vaccines and immunizations, or shots, before you travel. Find out what shot you need for where you are going, and make sure you get the right shots on time.

- Follow your healthy eating plan as much as possible when you eat out. Always carry a snack with you in case you have to wait for a waiter to serve you.

- Limit alcoholic beverages. Ask your healthcare team how many alcoholic beverages you can safely drink. Eat something when you drink to prevent low blood glucose.

- If you are taking a long trip by car, check your blood glucose levels before driving. Stop and check your blood glucose levels every two hours.

- Always carry your diabetes medicines and supplies in the car where you can reach them in case your blood glucose levels drop too low.

- In case you cannot leave for home on time, bring twice the amount of diabetes supplies and medicines you normally need.

- Take comfortable, well-fitting shoes on vacation. You will probably be walking more than usual. Keep your medical insurance card, emergency phone numbers, and a first aid kit handy.

- Wear or carry an identification tag or card that says you have diabetes.

- If you are going to be away for a long time, ask your doctor for a written prescription for your diabetes medicines and the name of a doctor in the place you are going to visit.

- Do not count on buying extra supplies when you are traveling, especially if you are going to another country. Different countries use different kinds of diabetes medicines.

When You Are Flying on a Plane

These tips can help you when you are flying on a plane:

- Ask your healthcare team in advance how to adjust your medicines, especially your insulin, if you are traveling across time zones.

- Take a letter from your doctor stating you have diabetes. The letter should include a list of all the medical supplies and medicines you need on the plane. In the letter, the doctor should also include a list of any devices that should not go through an X-ray machine.

- Carry your diabetes medicines and your blood testing supplies with you on the plane. Never put these items in your checked baggage.

- Bring food for meals and snacks on the plane.

- If you use an insulin pump, ask airport security to check the device by hand. X-ray machines can damage insulin pumps, whether the pump is on your body or in your luggage.

- When on a plane, get up from your seat and walk around when possible.

Action Steps If You Take Insulin

When you travel:

- Take a special insulated bag to carry your insulin to keep it from freezing or getting too hot.
- Bring extra supplies for taking insulin and testing your blood glucose levels in case of loss or breakage.
- Ask your doctor for a letter saying you have diabetes and need to carry supplies for taking insulin and testing blood glucose.

Action Steps If You Do Not Take Insulin

When you travel:

- Ask your healthcare team in advance how to adjust your medicines if you are traveling across time zones.
- Carry your diabetes medicines and your blood testing supplies with you on the plane.
- Ask your doctor for a letter saying you have diabetes and need to carry supplies for testing blood glucose.

When an Emergency or a Natural Disaster Happens

Everyone with diabetes should be prepared for emergencies and natural disasters, such as power outages or hurricanes. Always have a disaster kit ready. Include everything you need to take care of your diabetes, such as:

- A blood glucose meter, lancets, and testing strips
- Your diabetes medicines
- Insulin, syringes, and an insulated bag to keep insulin cool, if you take insulin
- A glucagon kit if you take insulin or if recommended by your doctor
- Glucose tablets and other food or drinks to treat low blood glucose
- Antibiotic cream or ointment
- A copy of your medical information, including a list of your conditions, medicines, and recent lab test results
- A list of your prescription names with dosage information and prescription numbers from your pharmacy

- Phone numbers for the American Red Cross (ARC) and other disaster relief groups

- You also might want to include some food that does not spoil, such as canned or dried food, along with bottled water

If You Are a Woman and Planning a Pregnancy

Keeping your blood glucose levels near normal before and during pregnancy helps protect both you and the fetus. Even before you become pregnant, your blood glucose levels should be close to the normal range.

Your healthcare team can work with you to get your blood glucose levels under control before you try to get pregnant. If you are already pregnant and you have diabetes, see your doctor right away. You can take steps to bring your blood glucose levels close to normal.

Your insulin needs may change when you are pregnant. Your doctor may want you to take more insulin and check your blood glucose levels more often.

Pregnancy Registries

Many women need to take medicine while they are pregnant. Some women take medicines for health problems, like diabetes or high blood pressure, that can start or get worse when a woman is pregnant. Some women use medicine before they find out they are pregnant.

A pregnancy exposure registry is a study that collects health information from women who take prescription medicines or vaccines when they are pregnant. Information is also collected on the newborn baby. This information is compared with women who have not taken medicine during pregnancy.

Enrolling in a pregnancy exposure registry can help improve safety information for medicines used during pregnancy and can be used to update drug labeling. If you would like your registry added to this list, please e-mail U.S. Food and Drug Administration (FDA) at Registries@fda.hhs.gov

(Source: "Pregnancy Registries," U.S. Department of Food and Drug Administration (FDA).)

If you plan to have a baby:

- Work with your healthcare team to get your blood glucose levels as close to the normal range as possible.

- See a doctor who has experience taking care of pregnant women with diabetes.

- Do not smoke, drink alcoholic beverages, or use harmful drugs.

- Follow your healthy eating plan.

Be sure to have your eyes, heart and blood vessels, blood pressure, and kidneys checked. Your doctor should also check for nerve damage. Pregnancy can make some health problems worse.

Chapter 40

Managing Diabetes in the Heat

Did you know that people who have diabetes—both type 1 and type 2—feel the heat more than people who do not have diabetes? Some reasons why:

- Certain diabetes complications, such as damage to blood vessels and nerves, can affect your sweat glands so your body cannot cool as effectively. That can lead to heat exhaustion and heat stroke, which is a medical emergency.

- People with diabetes get dehydrated (lose too much water from their bodies) more quickly. Not drinking enough liquids can raise blood sugar, and high blood sugar can make you urinate more, causing dehydration. Some commonly used medicines like diuretics ("water pills" to treat high blood pressure) can dehydrate you, too.

- High temperatures can change how your body uses insulin. You may need to test your blood sugar more often and adjust your insulin dose and what you eat and drink.

It Is the Heat and the Humidity

Even when it does not seem very hot outside, the combination of heat and humidity (moisture in the air) can be dangerous. When sweat evaporates (dries) on your skin, it removes heat and cools you. It is harder to stay cool in high humidity because sweat cannot evaporate as well.

Whether you are working out or just hanging out, it is a good idea to check the heat index—a measurement that combines temperature and humidity. Take steps to stay cool when

About This Chapter: This chapter includes text excerpted from "Managing Diabetes in the Heat," Centers for Disease Control and Prevention (CDC), July 12, 2018.

it reaches 80°F in the shade with 40 percent humidity or above. Important to know: The heat index can be up to 15°F higher in full sunlight, so stick to the shade when the weather warms up.

Physical activity is key to managing diabetes, but do not get active outdoors during the hottest part of the day or when the heat index is high. Get out early in the morning or in the evening when temperatures are lower, or go to an air-conditioned mall or gym to get active.

Summer Checklist
- Drink plenty of water.
- Test your blood sugar often.
- Keep medicines, supplies, and equipment out of the heat.
- Stay inside in air-conditioning when it is hottest.
- Wear loose, light clothing.
- Get medical attention for heat-related illness.
- Make a plan in case you lose power.
- Have a go-bag ready for emergencies.

Your Blood Sugar Knows Best

Kids out of school, vacations, get-togethers, family reunions. The summer season can throw off your routine, and possibly your diabetes management plan. Check your blood sugar more often to make sure it is in your target range no matter what the summer brings. It is especially important to recognize what low blood sugar feels like and treat it as soon as possible.

Warm-Weather Wisdom

- Drink plenty of water—even if you are not thirsty—so you do not get dehydrated.

- Avoid alcohol and drinks with caffeine, such as coffee and energy or sports drinks. They can lead to water loss and spike your blood sugar levels.

- Check your blood sugar before, during, and after you are active. You may need to change how much insulin you use. Ask your doctor if you would like help in adjusting your dosage.

- Wear loose-fitting, lightweight, and light-colored clothing.

- Wear sunscreen and a hat when you are outside. Sunburn can raise your blood sugar levels.

- Do not go barefoot, even on the beach or at the pool.

- Use your air conditioner or go to an air-conditioned building or mall to stay cool. In very high heat, a room fan would not cool you enough.

Too Hot to Handle

Know what else feels the heat? Diabetes, supplies, and equipment:

- Do not store insulin or oral diabetes medicine in direct sunlight or in a hot car. Check package information about how high temperatures can affect insulin and other medicines.

- If you are traveling, keep insulin and other medicines in a cooler. Do not put insulin directly on ice or on a gel pack.

- Heat can damage your blood sugar monitor, insulin pump, and other diabetes equipment. Do not leave them in a hot car, by a pool, in direct sunlight, or on the beach. The same goes for supplies such as test strips.

But do not let the summer heat stop you from taking your diabetes medicine and supplies with you when you are out and about. You will need to be able to test your blood sugar and take steps if it is too high or too low. Just make sure to protect your diabetes gear from the heat.

Stormy Weather

June 1 marks the beginning of the hurricane season. Severe thunderstorms with hail, high winds, and tornadoes are more likely in warm weather, too. People with diabetes face extra challenges if a strong storm knocks out the power or they have to seek shelter away from home. Plan how you will handle medicine that needs refrigeration, such as insulin. And be prepared by packing an emergency go-bag—a supply kit you can grab quickly if you need to leave your home.

Chapter 41

Smoking and Diabetes

What Is Diabetes?

Diabetes is a group of diseases in which blood sugar levels are higher than normal. Most of the food a person eats is turned into glucose (a kind of sugar) for the body's cells to use for energy. The pancreas, an organ near the stomach, makes a hormone called "insulin" that helps glucose get into the body's cells. When you have diabetes, your body either doesn't make enough insulin or cannot use the insulin very well. Less glucose gets into the cells and instead builds up in the blood. There are different types of diabetes. Type 2 is the most common in adults and accounts for more than 90 percent of all diabetes cases. Fewer people have type 1 diabetes, which most often develops in children, adolescents, or young adults.

How Is Smoking Related to Diabetes?

We now know that smoking causes type 2 diabetes. In fact, smokers are 30 to 40 percent more likely to develop type 2 diabetes than nonsmokers. And people with diabetes who smoke are more likely than nonsmokers to have trouble with insulin dosing and with controlling their disease. The more cigarettes you smoke, the higher your risk for type 2 diabetes. No matter what type of diabetes you have, smoking makes your diabetes harder to control. If you have diabetes and you smoke, you are more likely to have serious health problems from diabetes. Smokers with diabetes have higher risks for serious complications, including:

- Heart and kidney disease

About This Chapter: This chapter includes text excerpted from "Smoking and Diabetes," Centers for Disease Control and Prevention (CDC), March 22, 2018.

- Poor blood flow in the legs and feet that can lead to infections, ulcers, and possible amputation (removal of a body part by surgery, such as toes or feet)

- Retinopathy (an eye disease that can cause blindness)

- Peripheral neuropathy (damaged nerves to the arms and legs that causes numbness, pain, weakness, and poor coordination)

How Can Diabetes Be Prevented?

Do not smoke. Smoking increases your chance of having type 2 diabetes. Lose weight if you are overweight or obese. Stay active. Physical activity can prevent or delay type 2 diabetes in adults who are at high risk for the disease.

Help for Quitting Smoking

The U.S. Food and Drug Administration (FDA) has approved the following seven medicines as safe and effective to help smokers quit:

- Five types of nicotine replacement therapy
  - Patch*
  - Gum*
  - Lozenge*
  - Inhaler
  - Nasal spray

Available without a prescription

- Two nonnicotine medications
  - Bupropion (marketed as Wellbutrin and Zyban)
  - Varenicline (marketed as Chantix)

(Source: "Dual Use of Tobacco Products," Centers for Disease Control and Prevention (CDC).)

How Is Diabetes Treated?

Diabetes treatment and management can include:

- A healthy diet and physical activity program

- Weight loss (if overweight or obese)

- Medicines to control blood sugar by helping the body use insulin better

- Insulin taken by injections or by using an insulin pump

- Patient education to address problem-solving and coping skills needed to help manage diabetes and its complications

- Medicines to control cholesterol and blood pressure

Chapter 42

If Your Friend or Family Member Has Diabetes

One of the best ways to predict how well someone will manage their diabetes is how much support they get from family and friends.

Daily diabetes care is a lot to handle, from taking medicines, injecting insulin, and checking blood sugar levels to eating healthy food, being physically active, and keeping healthcare appointments. Your support can help make the difference between your friend or family member feeling overwhelmed or empowered.

What You Can Do

- **Learn about diabetes.** Find out why and when blood sugar should be checked, how to recognize and handle highs and lows (more below), what lifestyle changes are needed, and where to go for information and help.

- **Know that diabetes is individual.** Each person who has diabetes is different, and their treatment plan needs to be customized to their specific needs. It may be very different from that of other people you know with diabetes.

- **Ask** your friend or relative how you can help, and then listen to what they say. They may want reminders and assistance (or may not), and their needs can change over time.

- **Go to appointments** if it is okay with your relative or friend. You could learn more about how diabetes affects them and how you can be most helpful.

About This Chapter: This chapter includes text excerpted from "Friends, Family, and Diabetes," Centers for Disease Control and Prevention (CDC), August 7, 2018.

- **Give them time** in the daily schedule so they can manage their diabetes—check blood sugar, make healthy food, take a walk.

- **Avoid blame.** Many people with type 2 diabetes are overweight, but being overweight is just one of several factors involved. And blood sugar levels can be hard to control even with a healthy diet and regular physical activity. Diabetes is complicated.

- **Step back.** You may share the same toothpaste, but your family members may not want to share everything about managing diabetes with you. The same goes for a friend with diabetes.

- **Accept the ups and downs.** Moods can change with blood sugar levels, from happy to sad to irritable. It might just be the diabetes talking, but ask your friend or relative to tell their healthcare team if they feel sad on most days—it could be depression.

- **Be encouraging.** Tell them you know how hard they are trying. Remind them of their successes. Point out how proud you are of their progress.

- **Walk the talk.** Follow the same healthy food and fitness plan as your loved one; it is good for your health too. Lifestyle changes become habits more easily when you make them together.

- **Know the lows.** Hypoglycemia (low blood sugar) can be serious and needs to be treated immediately. Symptoms vary, so be sure to know your friend's or relative's specific signs, which could include:

  - Shakiness

  - Nervousness or anxiety

  - Sweating, chills, or clamminess

  - Irritability or impatience

  - Dizziness and difficulty concentrating

  - Hunger or nausea

  - Blurred vision

  - Weakness or fatigue

  - Anger, stubbornness, or sadness

- If your family member or friend has hypoglycemia several times a week, suggest that she or he talk with her or his healthcare team to see if the treatment plan needs to be adjusted.

- Offer to help them connect with other people who share their experiences. Online resources, such as the American Association of Diabetes Educators (AADE) Diabetes Online Community, or in-person diabetes support groups are good ways to get started.

Older Adults

Diabetes is more common in older adults, and it can be harder for them to manage. Older people may not be as able to notice high or low blood sugar levels, so it is especially important for you to know the signs and how it should be handled. They may have several diabetes complications, such as vision problems, kidney disease, or nerve damage, so regular appointments with their healthcare team are essential.

Better Together

The most important thing is the quality of life, yours and theirs. Sure, there will be highs and lows—blood sugar and otherwise—but together you can help make diabetes a part of life, instead of life feeling like it is all about diabetes.

Part Five
Nutrition, Physical Activity, and Weight Management

Chapter 43

Healthy Eating for Diabetics

If you have diabetes, eating healthy can help control your blood sugar. A diabetes-friendly diet means choosing healthy foods and sticking to regular mealtimes. In fact, a diabetes diet is the best eating plan for almost everyone. Some simple ways to build your own healthy eating plan include:

Eat Three Meals a Day

If you have diabetes, try to eat your meals at the same time each day. This helps your body better use the insulin it produces. In food, carbohydrates have the greatest effect on blood sugar levels. It is helpful to be aware of portion sizes.

A great way to control your food portions is with the plate method:

- Fill one half of your plate with non-starchy vegetables.
- Fill a quarter of your plate with grains and starchy foods.
- Fill a quarter of your plate with protein, such as baked, broiled, or grilled lean meats.
- Choose a small glass of low-fat milk or yogurt and a piece of fruit.

Try Non-Starchy Vegetables

Non-starchy vegetables are a great addition to any healthy meal. They are low in carbohydrates and high in fiber. The fiber can help to regulate blood sugars by slowing down digestion. Some non-starchy vegetables include:

- Asparagus

About This Chapter: This chapter includes text excerpted from "Healthy Eating for Diabetics," U.S. Department of Veterans Affairs (VA), March 11, 2019.

- Beets

- Broccoli

- Brussel

- Cabbage

- Carrots

- Cauliflower

- Celery

- Cucumbers

- Green Beans

- Lettuce

- Onions

- Sprouts

- Spinach

- Tomato Juice

- Tomatoes

- Yellow Squash

- Zucchini

When Should I Eat If I Have Diabetes?

Some people with diabetes need to eat at about the same time each day. Others can be more flexible with the timing of their meals. Depending on your diabetes medicines or type of insulin, you may need to eat the same amount of carbohydrates at the same time each day. If you take "mealtime" insulin, your eating schedule can be more flexible.

If you use certain diabetes medicines or insulin and you skip or delay a meal, your blood glucose level can drop too low. Ask your healthcare team when you should eat and whether you should eat before and after physical activity.

(Source: "Diabetes Diet, Eating, and Physical Activity," National Institute of Diabetes and Digestive and Kidney Diseases (NIDDK).)

Eat More Fiber and Less Carbohydrates

Eating fewer carbohydrates and adding fiber to your diet can help keep your blood sugar levels stable. To get more fiber in your diet, eat at least five servings of fruits and vegetables a day. You can also eat whole grains, beans, or legumes to increase your fiber intake. Cut down on carbohydrates by managing portion sizes with these foods:

- Starchy vegetables (potatoes, corn, peas)
- Beans and lentils
- Bread, cereal, pasta, rice
- Milk, yogurt, pudding
- Fruit and fruit juice
- Desserts, candy, ice cream, doughnuts, sugar-sweetened beverages

Talk with a registered dietitian nutritionist to learn how many carbohydrates you should eat every day. Be sure to check the Nutrition Facts label on the food packaging to find the nutrition content in foods.

Limit Your Sweets and Alcohol

A diabetes-friendly diet requires you to eat less candy, desserts, and fruit juice. Drinking alcohol can also affect your blood sugar levels, so only use alcohol with the permission of your doctor. To lower your intake of sugar, consider using sugar substitutes, and choose beverages such as diet soda, water, or unsweetened tea.

Strive for a Healthy Weight

A small amount of weight loss can improve blood sugar control. Food choices and portions can make a big difference in your success with eating healthy for diabetes and weight loss. Try reducing your portions, and learn to build a healthy plate.

Track Your Meals

For more information about eating healthy with diabetes, ask your healthcare provider to schedule an appointment for you to meet with a registered dietitian nutritionist. You and a dietitian can create a diabetes meal plan that meets your lifestyle and health needs.

What Other Foods and Drinks Should I Limit If I Have Diabetes?

Foods and drinks to limit include:

- Fried foods and other foods high in saturated fat and trans fat
- Foods high in salt, also called sodium
- Beverages with added sugars, such as juice, regular soda, and regular sports or energy drinks

Drink water instead of sweetened beverages. Consider using a sugar substitute in your coffee or tea.

If you drink alcohol, drink moderately—no more than one drink a day if you are a woman or two drinks a day if you are a man. If you use insulin or diabetes medicines that increase the amount of insulin your body makes, alcohol can make your blood glucose level drop too low. This is especially true if you have not eaten in a while. It is best to eat some food when you drink alcohol.

(Source: "Diabetes Diet, Eating, and Physical Activity," National Institute of Diabetes and Digestive and Kidney Diseases (NIDDK).)

Chapter 44

Making Healthy Food Choices

When you have diabetes, deciding what, when, and how much to eat may seem challenging. So, what can you eat, and how can you fit the foods you love into your meal plan? Eating healthy food at home and choosing healthy food when eating out are important in managing your diabetes.

The first step is to work with your doctor or dietitian to make a meal plan just for you. As soon as you find out you have diabetes, ask for a meeting with your doctor or dietitian to discuss how to make and follow a meal plan. During this meeting, you will learn how to choose healthier foods—a variety of vegetables and fruits, whole grains, fat-free or low-fat dairy foods, lean meats, and other proteins. You will also learn to watch your portion sizes and what to drink while staying within your calorie, fat, and carbohydrate (carb) limits.

You can still enjoy food while eating healthy. But how do you do that? Here are a few tips to help you when eating at home and away from home.

Eating Healthy Portions

An easy way to know portion sizes is to use the "plate method." Looking at your basic nine-inch dinner plate, draw an imaginary line down the middle of the plate, and divide one side in half.

- Fill the largest section with non-starchy vegetables, such as a salad, green beans, broccoli, cauliflower, cabbage, and carrots.

About This Chapter: This chapter includes text excerpted from "Diabetes—Eat Well," Centers for Disease Control and Prevention (CDC), March 20, 2019.

- In one of the smaller sections, put a grain or starchy food, such as bread, noodles, rice, corn, or potatoes.

- In the other smaller section, put your protein, such as fish, chicken, lean beef, tofu, or cooked dried beans.

Eating Out

American adults eat out at least three times a week on average. Restaurant portion sizes and how foods are prepared will affect the management of your diabetes. How can you eat out, manage your diabetes, and follow your meal plan? Here are some ideas.

- Talk to the server before you order. Do not be shy about asking questions about the food and, if it is not obvious, ask how foods are prepared.

- Choose meat or fish dishes that are baked, broiled, grilled, or poached instead of fried.

- If you see that portions are large, ask your server at the beginning of the meal to box half of your meal to-go and only serve the other half.

- Look at the menu for meals that are lower in fat or calories; many restaurants will mark healthier items.

- Remember that sugar-sweetened drinks can be a major source of calories. For low-calorie options, drink water, low-fat milk, unsweetened tea, black coffee, or diet drinks.

- If you drink alcohol, women should have no more than one drink per day. Men should have no more than two drinks per day. Avoid high-calorie mixed drinks.

- Skip dessert or share one with a friend. Or choose fruit for dessert. It will save calories and money.

Quick Tips

- Ask if the meat could be grilled or broiled instead of fried.
- Ask about dishes that are made with more vegetables.
- Ask if soups are creamy or broth-based. Broth-based soup is healthier.
- Ask that salad dressings/sauces be served on the side. Then only use a small amount.
- Think about splitting a dish with a friend.

Grocery Shopping

When you go grocery shopping, you are surrounded by foods and drinks that have a lot of fat, sugar, and salt. Avoid impulse buying; make a checklist of foods in your meal plan before you shop to help you focus on healthy foods for you and your family. Here are a few things to keep in mind.

- Your cart should look like the plate method above.

- Half of your food items should be non-starchy vegetables, such as lettuce, asparagus, broccoli, cauliflower, cucumber, spinach, mushrooms, onions, and peppers.

- The rest of the cart should have lean proteins, whole grains, fruit, dairy, beans, and starchy vegetables, such as corn, peas, parsnips, potatoes, pumpkin, squash, zucchini, and yams.

- You may be able to have a treat occasionally (check with your dietitian if you are unsure). Instead of treats high in calories, fat, and sugar, consider buying a healthier option, such as fruit, as a treat.

Try to stay in the outside aisles where stores usually have fruits, vegetables, meat, fish, and dairy. Spend less time in the inside aisles.

Quick Tips
- Do not go to the store or market hungry.
- Make a list before going to the store.
- Do not purchase items that are not in your meal plan.
- If you have favorite foods, discuss with your dietitian how to manage eating them occasionally.
- While at the store, do not linger in aisles with tempting foods.

Checking Labels on Packaged Foods

One way to make sure you are buying packaged foods that are lower in calories, sugar, and fat is to look at the updated Nutrition Facts label. Some of the information you will find is:

- Look at serving size first. It gives you important information for understanding the rest of the label. On the label in Figure 44.1, all the other numbers are for a 1½ cup serving. So, a 1½ cup of this food has 240 calories and 4 grams of total fat.

- The top of the label also lists how many servings are in a package. For example, this label is for a package with two servings. If you eat the whole package, you will have eaten twice as many calories, carbs, fats, and other nutrients as are listed on the label.
- Total carbohydrate on the label includes all types of carbs—sugar, starch, and fiber.
- Choose foods with lower calories, saturated fat, *trans* fat, added sugars, and sodium. These numbers are listed near the top of the label.
- Try to choose foods with more dietary fiber, which is listed lower on the label under total carbohydrates.

Nutrition Facts	
2 servings per container	
Serving size 1 1/2 cup (208g)	
Amount per serving	
Calories	**240**
	% Daily Value*
Total Fat 4g	**5%**
Saturated Fat 1.5g	**8%**
Trans Fat 0g	
Cholesterol 5mg	**2%**
Sodium 430mg	**19%**
Total Carbohydrate 46g	**17%**
Dietary Fiber 7g	**25%**
Total Sugars 4g	
Includes 2g Added Sugars	**4%**
Protein 11g	
Vitamin D 2mcg	10%
Calcium 260mg	20%
Iron 6mg	35%
Potassium 240mg	6%

* The % Daily Value (DV) tells you how much a nutrient in a serving of food contributes to a daily diet. 2,000 calories a day is used for general nutrition advice.

Figure 44.1. Nutrition Facts Label

Special Diet: Diabetes and Chronic Kidney Disease

About one in three American adults with diabetes also has chronic kidney disease (CKD). Diabetes and CKD diets share a lot of the same foods, but there are some important differences. Figuring out what to eat can be confusing.

The first and most important step is to meet with a registered dietitian who is trained in both diabetes and CKD nutrition. Together you will create a kidney-friendly plan that keeps blood sugar steady and fits in with your lifestyle.

Healthy Eating on Holidays and Special Occasions

For people with diabetes (and everyone else), the holiday season and special occasions add many temptations. Do not deprive yourself. You just have to plan ahead. Find ideas to help you plan for the holiday season and special occasions in tip sheets from the National Diabetes Education Program and the American Association for Diabetes Educators, which also has tips for healthy eating during big games and summer gatherings.

Chapter 45

Meal Plans and Diabetes

What Foods Can I Eat If I Have Diabetes?

You may worry that having diabetes means going without the foods you enjoy. The good news is that you can still eat your favorite foods, but you might need to eat smaller portions or enjoy them less often. Your healthcare team will help create a diabetes meal plan for you that meets your needs and likes.

The key to eating with diabetes is to eat a variety of healthy foods from all food groups, in the amounts your meal plan outlines.

The food groups are:

- **Vegetables**
  - Non-starchy: includes broccoli, carrots, greens, peppers, and tomatoes
  - Starchy: includes potatoes, corn, and green peas
- **Fruits**—includes oranges, melon, berries, apples, bananas, and grapes
- **Grains**—at least half of your grains for the day should be whole grains.
  - Includes wheat, rice, oats, cornmeal, barley, quinoa, bread, pasta, cereal, and tortillas
- **Protein**
  - Lean meat
  - Chicken or turkey without the skin

About This Chapter: This chapter includes text excerpted from "Diabetes Diet, Eating, and Physical Activity," National Institute of Diabetes and Digestive and Kidney Diseases (NIDDK), November 2016.

- Fish

- Eggs

- Nuts and peanuts

- Dried beans and certain peas, such as chickpeas and split peas

- Meat substitutes, such as tofu

- **Dairy**—nonfat or low fat

  - Milk or lactose-free milk if you have lactose intolerance

  - Yogurt

  - Cheese

Eat foods with heart-healthy fats, which mainly come from these foods:

- Oils that are liquid at room temperature, such as canola and olive oil

- Nuts and seeds

- Heart-healthy fish, such as salmon, tuna, and mackerel

- Avocado

Use oils when cooking food instead of butter, cream, shortening, lard, or stick margarine.

What Foods and Drinks Should I Limit If I Have Diabetes?

Foods and drinks to limit include:

- Fried foods and other foods high in saturated fat and trans fat

- Foods high in salt, also called "sodium"

- Sweets, such as baked goods, candy, and ice cream

- Beverages with added sugars, such as juice, regular soda, and regular sports or energy drinks

Drink water instead of sweetened beverages. Consider using a sugar substitute in your coffee or tea.

If you drink alcohol, drink moderately—no more than one drink a day if you are a woman or two drinks a day if you are a man. If you use insulin or diabetes medicines that increase the amount of insulin your body makes, alcohol can make your blood glucose level drop too low. This is especially true if you have not eaten in a while. It is best to eat some food when you drink alcohol.

When Should I Eat If I Have Diabetes?

Some people with diabetes need to eat at about the same time each day. Others can be more flexible with the timing of their meals. Depending on your diabetes medicines or type of insulin, you may need to eat the same amount of carbohydrates at the same time each day. If you take "mealtime" insulin, your eating schedule can be more flexible.

If you use certain diabetes medicines or insulin and you skip or delay a meal, your blood glucose level can drop too low. Ask your healthcare team when you should eat and whether you should eat before and after physical activity.

Timing Your Meals

When it comes to blood sugar control, when you eat is as important as what you eat. You may need to eat several small meals spaced evenly throughout the day to stay in your target range. So do not skip breakfast or wait until late in the day to get most of your calories. Doing so can cause your blood sugar to rise too high or fall too low.

(Source: "Diabetes: Meal Planning," Veterans Health Library, U.S. Department of Veterans Affairs (VA).)

How Much Can I Eat If I Have Diabetes?

Eating the right amount of food will also help you manage your blood glucose level and your weight. Your healthcare team can help you figure out how much food and how many calories you should eat each day.

Weight-Loss Planning

If you are overweight or have obesity, work with your healthcare team to create a weight-loss plan.

To lose weight, you need to eat fewer calories and replace less healthy foods with foods lower in calories, fat, and sugar.

If you have diabetes, are overweight or obese, and are planning to have a baby, you should try to lose any excess weight before you become pregnant.

Meal Plan Methods

Two common ways to help you plan how much to eat if you have diabetes are the plate method and carbohydrate counting, also called "carb counting." Check with your healthcare team about the method that is best for you.

Plate Method

The plate method helps you control your portion sizes. You do not need to count calories. The plate method shows the amount of each food group you should eat. This method works best for lunch and dinner.

Use a nine-inch plate. Put non-starchy vegetables on half of the plate, a meat or other protein on one-fourth of the plate, and a grain or other starch on the last one-fourth. Starches include starchy vegetables, such as corn and peas. You also may eat a small bowl of fruit or a piece of fruit, and drink a small glass of milk as included in your meal plan.

You can find many different combinations of food and more details about using the plate method from the American Diabetes Association's (ADA) Create Your Plate online.

Your daily eating plan also may include small snacks between meals.

Portion Sizes

You can use everyday objects or your hand to judge the size of a portion.

- 1 serving of meat or poultry is the palm of your hand or a deck of cards
- 1 3-ounce serving of fish is a checkbook
- 1 serving of cheese is six dice
- ½ cup of cooked rice or pasta is a rounded handful or a tennis ball
- 1 serving of a pancake or waffle is a DVD
- 2 tablespoons of peanut butter is a ping-pong ball

Carbohydrate Counting

Carbohydrate counting involves keeping track of the amount of carbohydrates you eat and drink each day. Because carbohydrates turn into glucose in your body, they affect your blood glucose level more than other foods do. Carb counting can help you manage your blood glucose level. If you take insulin, counting carbohydrates can help you know how much insulin to take.

The right amount of carbohydrates varies by how you manage your diabetes, including how physically active you are and what medicines you take, if any. Your healthcare team can help you create a personal eating plan based on carbohydrate counting.

The amount of carbohydrates in foods is measured in grams. To count carbohydrate grams in what you eat, you will need to:

- Learn which foods have carbohydrates.

- Read the Nutrition Facts food label, or learn to estimate the number of grams of carbohydrate in the foods you eat.

- Add the grams of carbohydrate from each food you eat to get your total for each meal and for the day.

Most carbohydrates come from starches, fruits, milk, and sweets. Try to limit carbohydrates with added sugars or those with refined grains, such as white bread and white rice. Instead, eat carbohydrates from fruits, vegetables, whole grains, beans, and low-fat or nonfat milk.

In addition to using the plate method and carb counting, you may want to visit a registered dietitian (RD) for medical nutrition therapy.

Chapter 46

Carbohydrate Counting

What Is Carbohydrate Counting?

Carbohydrate counting, also called "carb counting," is a meal planning tool for people with type 1 or type 2 diabetes. Carbohydrate counting involves keeping track of the amount of carbohydrate in the foods you eat each day.

Carbohydrates are one of the main nutrients found in food and drinks. Protein and fat are the other main nutrients. Carbohydrates include sugars, starches, and fiber. Carbohydrate counting can help you control your blood glucose, also called "blood sugar," levels because carbohydrates affect your blood glucose more than other nutrients.

Healthy carbohydrates, such as whole grains, fruits, and vegetables, are an important part of a healthy eating plan because they can provide both energy and nutrients, such as vitamins, minerals, and fiber. Fiber can help you prevent constipation, lower your cholesterol levels, and control your weight.

Unhealthy carbohydrates are often food and drinks with added sugars. Although unhealthy carbohydrates can also provide energy, they have little to no nutrients.

The amount of carbohydrate in foods is measured in grams. To count the grams of carbohydrate in the foods you eat, you will need to:

- Know which foods contain carbohydrates.

- Learn to estimate the number of grams of carbohydrate in the foods you eat.

About This Chapter: This chapter includes text excerpted from "Carbohydrate Counting and Diabetes," National Institute of Diabetes and Digestive and Kidney Diseases (NIDDK), June 2014. Reviewed June 2019.

- Add up the number of grams of carbohydrate from each food you eat to get your total for the day.

Your doctor can refer you to a dietitian or diabetes educator who can help you develop a healthy eating plan based on carbohydrate counting.

Which Foods Contain Carbohydrates

Foods that contain carbohydrates include:

- Grains, such as bread, noodles, pasta, crackers, cereals, and rice

- Fruits, such as apples, bananas, berries, mangoes, melons, and oranges

- Dairy products, such as milk and yogurt

- Legumes, including dried beans, lentils, and peas

- Snack foods and sweets, such as cakes, cookies, candy, and other desserts

- Juices, soft drinks, fruit drinks, sports drinks, and energy drinks that contain sugars

- Vegetables, especially starchy vegetables, such as potatoes, corn, and peas

Potatoes, peas, and corn are called "starchy vegetables" because they are high in starch. These vegetables have more carbohydrates per serving than non-starchy vegetables.

Examples of non-starchy vegetables are asparagus, broccoli, carrots, celery, green beans, lettuce and other salad greens, peppers, spinach, tomatoes, and zucchini.

Foods that do not contain carbohydrates include meat, fish, and poultry; most types of cheese; nuts; and oils and other fats.

What Happens When I Eat Foods Containing Carbohydrates

When you eat foods containing carbohydrates, your digestive system breaks down the sugars and starches into glucose. Glucose is one of the simplest forms of sugar. Glucose then enters your bloodstream from your digestive tract and raises your blood glucose levels. The hormone insulin, which comes from the pancreas or from insulin shots, helps cells throughout your body absorb glucose and use it for energy. Once glucose moves out of the blood into cells, your blood glucose levels go back down.

How Can Carbohydrate Counting Help Me?

Carbohydrate counting can help keep your blood glucose levels close to normal. Keeping your blood glucose levels as close to normal as possible may help you:

- Stay healthy longer

- Prevent or delay diabetes problems, such as kidney disease, blindness, nerve damage, and blood vessel disease that can lead to heart attacks, strokes, and amputations—surgery to remove a body part

- Feel better and more energetic

You may also need to take diabetes medicines or have insulin shots to control your blood glucose levels. Discuss your blood glucose targets with your doctor. Targets are numbers you aim for. To meet your targets, you will need to balance your carbohydrate intake with physical activity and diabetes medicines or insulin shots.

How Much Carbohydrate Do I Need Each Day?

The daily amount of carbohydrate, protein, and fat for people with diabetes has not been defined—what is best for one person may not be best for another. Everyone needs to get enough carbohydrate to meet the body's needs for energy, vitamins and minerals, and fiber.

Experts suggest that carbohydrate intake for most people should be between 45 and 65 percent of their total calories. People on low-calorie diets and people who are physically inactive may want to aim for the lower end of that range.

One gram of carbohydrate provides about 4 calories, so you will have to divide the number of calories you want to get from carbohydrates by 4 to get the number of grams. For example, if you want to eat 1,800 total calories per day and get 45 percent of your calories from carbohydrates, you would aim for about 200 grams of carbohydrate daily. You would calculate that amount as follows:

- 0.45 x 1,800 calories = 810 calories

- 810 ÷ 4 = 202.5 grams of carbohydrate

You will need to spread out your carbohydrate intake throughout the day. A dietitian or diabetes educator can help you learn what foods to eat, how much to eat, and when to eat based on your weight, activity level, medicines, and blood glucose targets.

How Can I Find Out How Much Carbohydrate Is in the Foods I Eat?

You will need to learn to estimate the amount of carbohydrate in foods you typically eat. For example, the following amounts of carbohydrate-rich foods each contain about 15 grams of carbohydrate:

- One slice of bread

- One 6-inch tortilla

- ⅓ cup of pasta

- ⅓ cup of rice

- ½ cup of canned fruit; fresh fruit; fruit juice; or one small piece of fresh fruit, such as a small apple or orange

- ½ cup of pinto beans

- ½ cup of starchy vegetables, such as mashed potatoes, cooked corn, peas, or lima beans

- ¾ cup of dry cereal or ½ cup cooked cereal

- 1 tablespoon of jelly

Some foods are so low in carbohydrates that you may not have to count them unless you eat large amounts. For example, most non-starchy vegetables are low in carbohydrates. A ½-cup serving of cooked non-starchy vegetables or a cup of raw vegetables has only about five grams of carbohydrate.

As you become familiar with which foods contain carbohydrates and how many grams of carbohydrate are in food you eat, carbohydrate counting will be easier.

Nutrition Labels

You can find out how many grams of carbohydrate are in the foods you eat by checking the nutrition labels on food packages. Following is an example of a nutrition label:

Nutrition labels tell you:

- The food's serving size—such as one slice or a ½ cup

- The total grams of carbohydrate per serving

- Other nutrition information, including calories and the amount of protein and fat per serving

Nutrition Facts

Serving Size 1 cup (228g)
Servings Per Container 2

Amount Per Serving

Calories 250   Calories from Fat 110

	% Daily Value*
Total Fat 12g	**18%**
Saturated Fat 3g	**15%**
Trans Fat 3g	
Cholesterol 30mg	**10%**
Sodium 470mg	**20%**
Total Carbohydrate 31g	**10%**
Dietary Fiber 0g	**0%**
Sugars 5g	
Protein 5g	

Vitamin A	**4%**
Vitamin C	**2%**
Calcium	**20%**
Iron	**4%**

* Percent Daily Values are based on a 2,000 calorie diet.
Your Daily Values may be higher or lower depending on
your calorie needs.

	Calories:	2,000	2,500
Total Fat	Less than	65g	80g
Sat Fat	Less than	20g	25g
Cholesterol	Less than	300mg	300mg
Sodium	Less than	2,400mg	2,400mg
Total Carbohydrate		300g	375g
Dietary Fiber		25g	30g

Figure 46.1. A Sample Nutrition Facts Label

If you have 2 servings instead of 1, such as 1 cup of pinto beans instead of a ½ cup, you multiply the number of grams of carbohydrate in 1 serving—for example, 15—by 2 to get the total number of grams of carbohydrate—30.

15 x 2 = 30

Cooking at Home

To find out the amount of carbohydrate in homemade foods, you will need to estimate and add up the grams of carbohydrate from the ingredients. You can use books or websites that list the typical carbohydrate content of homemade items to estimate the amount of carbohydrate in a serving.

You can also weigh foods with a scale or measure amounts with measuring cups or spoons to estimate the amount of carbohydrate. For example, if a nutrition label shows that 1½ cups of cereal contains 45 grams of carbohydrate, then ½ cup will have 15 grams of carbohydrate, and 1 cup will have 30 grams of carbohydrate.

Eating Out

Some restaurants provide nutrition information that lists grams of carbohydrate. You can also use carbohydrate counting food lists to estimate the amount of carbohydrate in restaurant meals.

Can I Eat Sweets and Other Foods and Drinks with Added Sugars?

Yes, you can eat sweets and other foods and drinks with added sugars. However, you should limit your intake of these high-carbohydrate foods and drinks because they are often high in calories and low in vitamins, minerals, and fiber. Fiber-rich whole grains, fruits, vegetables, and beans are wiser choices.

What Are Added Sugars?

Added sugars are various forms of sugar added to foods or drinks during processing or preparation. Naturally occurring sugars such as those in milk and fruits are not added sugars but are carbohydrates. The most common sources of added sugars for Americans are:

- Sugar-sweetened soft drinks, fruit drinks, sports drinks, and energy drinks
- Grain-based desserts, such as cakes, cookies, and doughnuts
- Milk-based desserts and products, such as ice cream, sweetened yogurt, and sweetened milk
- Candy

Reading the list of ingredients for foods and drinks can help you find added sugars, such as:

- Sugar, raw sugar, brown sugar, and invert sugar—a mixture of fructose and glucose
- Corn syrup and malt syrup
- High-fructose corn syrup, often used in soft drinks and juices
- Honey, molasses, and agave nectar
- Dextrose, fructose, glucose, lactose, and sucrose

For a healthier eating plan, limit foods and drinks with added sugars.

Instead of eating sweets every day, try eating them in small amounts once in a while so you do not fill up on foods that are low in nutrition. Ask your dietitian or diabetes educator about including sweets in your eating plan.

How Can I Tell Whether Carbohydrate Counting Is Working for Me?

Checking your blood glucose levels can help you tell whether carbohydrate counting is working for you. You can check your blood glucose levels using a glucose meter.

You should also have an A1C blood test at least twice a year. The A1C test reflects the average amount of glucose in your blood during the past three months.

If your blood glucose levels are too high, you may need to make changes in your eating plan or other lifestyle changes. For example, you may need to make wiser food choices, be more physically active, or make changes to your diabetes medicines. Talk with your doctor about what changes you need to make to control your blood glucose levels.

If you use an insulin pump or take more than one daily insulin shot, ask your doctor how to adjust your insulin when you eat something that is not in your usual eating plan.

Can I Use Carbohydrate Counting If I Am Pregnant?

You can use carbohydrate counting to help control your blood glucose levels when you are pregnant. Meeting your blood glucose targets during pregnancy is important for your health and your baby's health. High blood glucose during pregnancy can harm the baby and increase the baby's chances of having type 2 diabetes later in life.

Women diagnosed with gestational diabetes—a type of diabetes that develops only during pregnancy—can also use carbohydrate counting to help control their blood glucose levels.

Talk with your doctor about using carbohydrate counting to help meet your blood glucose targets during your pregnancy.

271

Chapter 47

Diabetes and Dietary Supplements

What the Science Says about the Effectiveness and Safety of Dietary Supplements for Diabetes
Alpha-Lipoic Acid

- Alpha-lipoic acid is being studied for its effect on complications of diabetes, including diabetic macular edema (an eye condition that can cause vision loss) and diabetic neuropathy (nerve damage caused by diabetes).

  - In a 2011 study of 235 people with type 2 diabetes, 2 years of supplementation with alpha-lipoic acid did not help to prevent macular edema.

  - A 2016 assessment of treatments for symptoms of diabetic neuropathy that included 2 studies of oral alpha-lipoic acid, with a total of 205 participants, indicated that alpha-lipoic acid may be helpful.

- Safety

  - High doses of alpha-lipoic acid supplements can cause stomach problems.

About This Chapter: Text under the heading "What the Science Says about the Effectiveness and Safety of Dietary Supplements for Diabetes?" is excerpted from "Diabetes and Dietary Supplements," National Center for Complementary and Integrative Health (NCCIH), May 30, 2018; Text under the heading "Six Things to Know about Type 2 Diabetes and Dietary Supplements" is excerpted from "6 Things to Know about Type 2 Diabetes and Dietary Supplements," National Center for Complementary and Integrative Health (NCCIH), July 21, 2017.

Chromium

- Found in many foods, chromium is an essential trace mineral. If you have too little chromium in your diet, your body cannot use glucose efficiently.

  - Taking chromium supplements, along with conventional care, slightly improved blood sugar control in people with diabetes (primarily type 2) who had poor blood sugar control, a 2014 review concluded. The review included 25 studies with about 1,600 participants.

- Safety

  - Chromium supplements may cause stomach pain and bloating, and there have been a few reports of kidney damage, muscular problems, and skin reactions following large doses. The effects of taking chromium long term have not been well investigated.

Herbal Supplements

- There is not any reliable evidence that any herbal supplements can help to control diabetes or its complications.

  - There are no clear benefits of cinnamon for people with diabetes.

  - Other herbal supplements studied for diabetes include bitter melon, various Chinese herbal medicines, fenugreek, ginseng, milk thistle, and sweet potato. Studies have not proven that any of these are effective, and some may have side effects.

- Safety

  - There is little conclusive information on the safety of herbal supplements for people with diabetes.

  - Cassia cinnamon, the most common type of cinnamon sold in the United States and Canada, contains varying amounts of a chemical called "coumarin," which might cause or worsen liver disease. In most cases, cassia cinnamon does not have enough coumarin to make you sick. However, for some people, such as those with liver disease, taking a large amount of cassia cinnamon might worsen their condition.

  - Using herbs, such as St. John's wort, prickly pear cactus, aloe, or ginseng, with conventional diabetes drugs can cause unwanted side effects.

Magnesium

- Found in many foods, including in high amounts in bran cereal, certain seeds and nuts, and spinach, magnesium is essential to the body's ability to process glucose.

  - Magnesium deficiency may increase the risk of developing diabetes. A number of studies have looked at whether taking magnesium supplements helps people who have diabetes or who are at risk of developing it. However, the studies are generally small, and their results are not conclusive.

- Safety

  - Large doses of magnesium in supplements can cause diarrhea and abdominal cramping. Very large doses—more than 5,000 mg per day—can be deadly.

Omega-3s

- Taking omega-3 fatty acid supplements, such as fish oil, has not been shown to help people who have diabetes control their blood sugar levels or reduce their risk of heart disease.

- Fish and other seafood—especially cold-water fatty fish, such as salmon and tuna—contain omega-3 fatty acids. Studies on the effects of eating fish have had conflicting results, according to two 2012 research reviews with hundreds of thousands of participants and a 2017 review. Some research from the United States and Europe found that people who ate more fish had a higher incidence of diabetes. Research from Asia and Australia found the opposite—eating more fish was associated with a lower risk of diabetes. There is no strong evidence explaining these differences.

- Safety

  - Omega-3 supplements do not usually have side effects. When side effects do occur, they typically consist of minor symptoms, such as bad breath, indigestion, or diarrhea.

  - Omega-3 supplements may interact with drugs that affect blood clotting.

Selenium

- An assessment of 4 studies involving more than 20,000 total participants found that selenium supplementation did not reduce the likelihood that people would develop type 2 diabetes.

- Safety

  - Long-term intake of too much selenium can have harmful effects, including hair and nail loss, gastrointestinal symptoms, and nervous system abnormalities.

Vitamins

- Studies generally show that taking vitamin C does not improve blood sugar control or other conditions in people with diabetes. However, a 2017 research review of 22 studies with 937 participants found weak evidence that vitamin C helped with blood sugar in people with type 2 diabetes when they took it for longer than 30 days.

- Having low levels of vitamin D is associated with an increased risk of developing a metabolic disorder, such as type 2 diabetes, metabolic syndrome, or insulin resistance, studies and research reviews from the past 5 years have found. However, taking vitamin D does not appear to help prevent diabetes or improve blood sugar levels for adults with normal levels, prediabetes, or type 2 diabetes, a 2014 research review of 35 studies with 43,407 participants showed.

- Safety

  - Taking too much vitamin D can cause nausea, constipation, weakness, kidney damage, disorientation, and problems with your heart rhythm. You are unlikely to get too much vitamin D from food or the sun.

Other Supplements

- The evidence is still very preliminary on how supplements or foods rich in polyphenols—antioxidants found in tea, coffee, wine, fruits, grains, and vegetables—might affect diabetes.

Nutrition and Physical Activity for People with Diabetes

Nutrition and physical activity are important parts of a healthy lifestyle for people with diabetes. Eating well and being physically active can help you:

- Keep your blood glucose level, blood pressure, and cholesterol in your target ranges
- Lose weight or stay at a healthy weight
- Prevent or delay diabetes problems
- Feel good and have more energy

Six Things to Know about Type 2 Diabetes and Dietary Supplements

Diabetes is a group of chronic diseases that affect metabolism—the way the body uses food for energy and growth. Millions of people have diabetes, which can lead to serious health problems if it is not managed well. Conventional medical treatments and following a healthy lifestyle, including watching your weight, can help you prevent, manage, and control many complications of diabetes. Researchers are studying several complementary health approaches, including dietary supplements, to see if they can help people manage type 2 diabetes or lower their risk of developing the disease; however, there is currently not enough scientific evidence to suggest that any dietary supplements can help prevent or manage type 2 diabetes.

Here are six things you should know about taking dietary supplements for type 2 diabetes:

1. A healthy diet, physical activity, and blood glucose testing are the basic tools for managing type 2 diabetes. Your healthcare providers will help you learn to manage your diabetes and track how well you are controlling it. It is very important not to replace proven conventional medical treatment for diabetes with an unproven health product or practice.

2. Some dietary supplements may have side effects, including interacting with your diabetes treatment or increasing your risk of kidney problems. This is of particular concern because diabetes is the leading cause of chronic kidney disease and kidney failure in the United States. Supplement use should be monitored closely in patients who have or are at risk for kidney disease.

3. Chromium (an essential trace mineral found in many foods) has been studied for preventing diabetes and controlling glucose levels, but research has found it has few or no benefits. There have been a few reports of kidney damage, muscular problems, and skin reactions following large doses of chromium.

4. There is mixed evidence that magnesium helps to manage diabetes—benefits of magnesium supplements on diabetes have been found in some, but not all clinical studies. However, research suggests that people with lower magnesium intake may have a greater risk of developing diabetes. A study found an association between a higher intake of cereal fiber and magnesium and a reduced risk of developing type 2 diabetes. Large doses of magnesium in supplements can cause diarrhea and abdominal cramping, and very large doses—more than 5,000 mg/day per day—can be deadly.

5. There is no strong evidence that herbs and other dietary supplements, including cinnamon, alpha-lipoic acid, and omega-3s, can help to control diabetes or its complications. Researchers have found some risks but no clear benefits of cinnamon for people with diabetes. For example, a 2012 review of the scientific literature did not support using cinnamon for type 1 or type 2 diabetes.

6. Talk with your healthcare provider before considering any dietary supplement for yourself, particularly if you are pregnant or nursing, or for a child. Do not replace scientifically proven treatments for diabetes with unproven health products or practices. The consequences of not following your prescribed medical regimen for diabetes can be very serious.

> Kidney disease has been linked to using some dietary supplements. This is of particular concern for people with diabetes, since diabetes is the leading cause of kidney disease. If you have or are at risk for kidney disease, a healthcare provider should closely monitor your use of supplements.

Chapter 48

Physical Activity and Diabetes

Physical activity is very important for people with diabetes. And, it is not as hard as you might think to be more active.

Being More Active Is Better for You

If you have diabetes, being active makes your body more sensitive to insulin (the hormone that allows cells in your body to use blood sugar for energy), which helps manage your diabetes. Physical activity also helps control blood sugar levels and lowers your risk of heart disease and nerve damage.

Some additional benefits include:

- Maintaining a healthy weight

- Losing weight, if needed

- Feeling happier

- Sleeping better

- Improving your memory

- Controlling your blood pressure

About This Chapter: This chapter includes text excerpted from "Diabetes—Get Active!" Centers for Disease Control and Prevention (CDC), April 24, 2018.

- Lowering low-density lipoprotein (LDL, "bad") cholesterol and raising high-density lipoprotein (HDL, "good") cholesterol

How to Benefit from Physical Activity

The goal is to get at least 150 minutes per week of moderate-intensity physical activity. One way to do this is to try to fit in at least 20 to 25 minutes of activity every day. Also, on 2 or more days a week, include activities that work all major muscle groups (legs, hips, back, abdomen, chest, shoulders, and arms).

Examples of moderate-intensity physical activities include:

- Walking briskly

- Doing housework

- Mowing the lawn

- Dancing

- Swimming

- Bicycling

- Playing sports

These activities work your large muscles, increase your heart rate, and make you breathe harder, which are important goals for fitness. Stretching helps to make you flexible and prevent soreness after being physically active.

Most kinds of physical activity can help you take care of your diabetes. Certain activities may be unsafe for some people, such as those with low vision or nerve damage to their feet. Ask your healthcare team what physical activities are safe for you. Many people choose walking with friends or family members for their activity.

Doing different types of physical activity each week will give you the most health benefits. Mixing it up also helps reduce boredom and lower your chance of getting hurt. Try these options for physical activity.

If you have been inactive or you are trying a new activity, start slowly, with 5 to 10 minutes a day. Then add a little more time each week.

(Source: "Diabetes Diet, Eating, and Physical Activity," National Institute of Diabetes and Digestive and Kidney Diseases (NIDDK).)

Ways to Get Started

- **Find something you like.** Exercising by doing something you enjoy is important because if you do not like it, you will not stick with it. Find an activity that you and your healthcare provider agree you can do regularly for the best results.

- **Start small.** If you are not already physically active, you should begin slowly and work your way up to the desired level. For example, you could park farther from the door, take the stairs, do yard work, or walk the dog. Start small and gradually add a little more time and intensity each week.

- **Pick a goal.** An example of a goal could be to walk a mile every day for a month or to be active every weekday for 30 minutes. Be specific and realistic. Always discuss your activity goals with your healthcare provider.

- **Schedule it in.** The more regular activity you do, the quicker it will become a habit. Think of ways to link activity to daily life. For example, you could schedule walking with a coworker after lunch. Try not to go more than two days in a row without being active.

Buddies with Benefits

When you work out with a partner, you are likely to:

Feel more motivated. When you and your buddy encourage each other, you will work harder (and get better results!). And there's nothing wrong with a little friendly competition.

Be more adventurous. It's easier to try new things with a buddy. You may just find an activity you love, one that feels more like fun and less like a workout.

Be more consistent. When someone else is counting on you to show up, you won't want to let them down.

To enjoy all those benefits, you will need the right workout buddy. Look for someone with the same goals, schedule, and commitment you have. Someone who makes you feel positive and inspires you to hit the trail or treadmill on a regular basis.

(Source: "Find the Right Workout Buddy," Centers for Disease Control and Prevention (CDC).)

Ways to Turn Excuses into Solutions

For every excuse, there is a workable solution. Listed below are some of the most common excuses and suggested solutions.

Table 48.1. Most Common Excuses and Suggested Solutions

I'm Not More Active Because	Ways to Make It Work
It's just too hard.	If you think being more active means hours at the gym, it's just not true! You can start by walking for 10 minutes after dinner, gradually building up to 30 minutes most days.
The results take too long.	Some benefits start right away, even if they don't seem obvious to you. Check your blood sugar before and after you take a walk. You'll likely see a lower number after the walk. If you stick with it over time (weeks, months, years), you will see more obvious results.
It's just not fun.	It can be lots of fun if you find an activity you enjoy. Don't force yourself to do something you don't like. You won't stick with it. Try doing a new activity a couple of times before deciding whether to continue with that activity. If one activity isn't a good fit, don't give up. Try something else.
It costs too much.	The costs for gym memberships and fitness classes can add up. However, walking during lunch or after dinner, dancing to your favorite tunes at home, or working out to online videos are free and can be done at times that are more convenient for you.
It's hard to find the time.	Find ways to squeeze physical activity into your day-to-day life. For example, take the stairs instead of the elevator, play outside with your children, get up and move during TV commercials. Try to fit in at least 20 to 25 minutes of activity every day, which will help it become a habit.
I'm just too old.	It's never too late to start being more active! Low-impact activities like pool walking and swimming are examples. Talk to your healthcare provider about activities that you can do to get started.
I'm too out of shape.	Start slowly, and work your way up to your desired level. Add simple activities to your daily life like walking to your mailbox, or when you're running errands park a little farther from the door. Discuss other ideas with your healthcare provider.

Special Considerations for People with Diabetes

Before starting any physical activity, check with your healthcare provider to talk about the best physical activities for you. Be sure to discuss which activities you like, how to prepare, and what you should avoid.

- Drink plenty of fluids while being physically active to prevent dehydration (harmful loss of water in the body).

- Make sure to check your blood sugar before being physically active, especially if you take insulin.

  - If it is below 100 mg/dL, you may need to eat a small snack containing 15 to 30 grams of carbohydrates, such as 2 tablespoons of raisins or ½ cup of fruit juice or regular soda (not diet), or glucose tablets so your blood sugar does not fall too low while being physically active. Low blood sugar (hypoglycemia) can be very serious.

  - If it is above 240 mg/dL, your blood sugar may be too high (hyperglycemia) to be active safely. Test your urine for ketones—substances made when your body breaks down fat for energy. The presence of ketones indicates that your body does not have enough insulin to control your blood sugar. If you are physically active when you have high ketone levels, you risk ketoacidosis—a serious diabetes complication that needs immediate treatment.

- When you are physically active, wear cotton socks and athletic shoes that fit well and are comfortable.

- After your activity, check to see how it has affected your blood glucose level.

- After being physically active, check your feet for sores, blisters, irritation, cuts, or other injuries. Call your healthcare provider if an injury does not begin to heal after two days.

Chapter 49

Stay at a Healthy Weight

When it comes to weight loss, there is no lack of fad diets promising fast results. But, such diets limit your nutritional intake, can be unhealthy, and tend to fail in the long run.

The key to achieving and maintaining a healthy weight is not about short-term dietary changes. It is about a lifestyle that includes healthy eating, regular physical activity, and balancing the number of calories you consume with the number of calories your body uses.

Staying in control of your weight contributes to good health now and as you age.

Why Is a Healthy Weight Important?

Reaching and maintaining a healthy weight is important for overall health and can help you prevent and control many diseases and conditions. If you are overweight or obese, you are at higher risk of developing serious health problems, including heart disease, high blood pressure, type 2 diabetes, gallstones, breathing problems, and certain cancers. That is why maintaining a healthy weight is so important: It helps you lower your risk for developing these problems, helps you feel good about yourself, and gives you more energy to enjoy life.

(Source: "Aim for a Healthy Weight," National Heart, Lung, and Blood Institute (NHLBI).)

About This Chapter: Text in this chapter begins with excerpts from "Healthy Weight," Centers for Disease Control and Prevention (CDC), October 2, 2018; Text under the heading "Weight and Exercise" is excerpted from "Stay Healthy," Centers for Disease Control and Prevention (CDC), April 6, 2018; Text under the heading "Tips for Successful Weight Loss" is excerpted from "Tips for Successful Weight Loss," Office on Women's Health (OWH), U.S. Department of Health and Human Services (HHS), March 14, 2019.

Weight and Exercise
How Does Maintaining a Healthy Body Weight Help People with Diabetes Stay Healthy?

Most people newly diagnosed with type 2 diabetes are overweight. Excess weight, particularly in the abdomen, makes it difficult for cells to respond to insulin, resulting in high blood glucose. Often, people with type 2 diabetes are able to lower their blood glucose by losing weight and increasing physical activity. Losing weight also helps lower the risk for other health problems that especially affect people with diabetes, such as heart disease.

How Does Exercise Help People with Diabetes Stay Healthy?

Physical activity can help you control your blood glucose, weight, and blood pressure, as well as raise your high-density lipoprotein (HDL, "good") cholesterol and lower your low-density lipoprotein (LDL, "bad") cholesterol. It also can help prevent heart and blood flow problems.

Experts recommend moderate-intensity physical activity for at least 30 minutes on five or more days of the week. Talk to your healthcare provider about a safe exercise plan. She or he may check your heart and your feet to be sure you have no special problems. If you have high blood pressure, eye, or foot problems you may need to avoid some kinds of exercise.

Tips for Successful Weight Loss

The key is to focus on small, healthy changes that you can stick with for the rest of your life. Losing weight is part of living a healthier lifestyle. Try some of these tips to help give you the best chance of success.

- **Set realistic goals that can be measured.** Do not expect to lose 30 pounds in the first month. Set a goal of 1 pound a week and track your progress. (Talk to your doctor or nurse to find out how much weight is safe for you to lose.) Reward yourself with a fun activity (but not an unhealthy treat) when you meet each goal!

- **Plan your meals ahead of time.** Most people who eat healthy plan most of their meals ahead of time so that they don't binge as much on unhealthy food. Figure out which meals you'll be eating at home for the week ahead. Make a grocery store list for those meals and snacks. Stick to your list when you go shopping.

- **Make just one change at a time.** It can be difficult to change everything you eat all at once. Pick one small healthy eating goal and work on that until you can reach that goal most of the time—or until you figure out why that goal will not work for you. Then pick another healthy eating goal.

- **Don't cut out all treats.** It's tempting to tell yourself that you'll stop eating all unhealthy foods (like cookies, cake, chips, soda, and French fries) in order to lose weight. This strategy may be easy at first, but it can be difficult to continue over time. You might end up binging on unhealthy foods because you feel deprived. Choose your treats ahead of time, cut back on the number of times you have unhealthy food, and keep the portion size small.

- **Choose smaller portions when eating out.** Restaurant foods are often high in salt, fat, and calories. Order the small or lower-calorie option, share a meal, or take home part of the meal. Calorie information may be available on menus, in a pamphlet, on food wrappers, or online.

- **Drink water first.** Sometimes what we think is hunger is actually thirst. Try drinking water before snacking to see if that helps you put off eating until it's time for a meal. Or maybe you will eat less if you've filled up on some water first.

- **Don't forget about calories from alcohol.** It can be difficult to know exactly how many calories are in a glass of wine or a mixed drink. If you drink alcohol and want to lose weight, cutting down on the number of drinks you have each week is one of the easiest ways to lose weight, since you don't get any essential vitamins, minerals, or other nutrients from alcohol.

- **Lift some weights.** Muscle burns more calories than fat. Aim for two or three strength-training sessions a week. Allow a day or so in between workouts for your body to rest.

- **Deal with stress.** Stress can make weight gain more likely. Find ways to unplug and lower stress that work for you. Some options include meditation, yoga, reading, religious worship, spending quality time with friends and family, learning a new healthy recipe, trying out a new physical activity like bicycling or an exercise class, or volunteering in your community.

- **Keep trying.** One of the keys to weight loss is to keep trying. If a certain strategy doesn't work for you, that doesn't mean you are a failure. As long as you learn something from that particular experience, it can give you valuable insight into what might work better for you in the future.

- **Try something different.** If you tried losing weight on your own in the past and it didn't work, try joining a weight-loss group. If your partner isn't willing to eat healthy

287

along with you, talk about how they might support you in the future. Figure out some of the reasons why you weren't able to lose weight before and do it differently next time. If you are still challenged, consider seeing a doctor who specializes in weight management.

Chapter 50

Early Weight-Loss Surgery May Improve Type 2 Diabetes and Blood Pressure Outcomes

Despite similar weight loss, teens who had gastric bypass surgery were significantly more likely to have remission of both type 2 diabetes and high blood pressure when compared to adults who had the same procedure. Results are from a National Institutes of Health (NIH)-funded study comparing outcomes in the two groups five years after surgery. Previously, no treatment has shown longer-term effectiveness at reversing type 2 diabetes in youth, which tends to advance more quickly than in adults.

Researchers evaluated 161 teens and 396 adults who underwent this surgery at clinical centers participating in Teen-Longitudinal Assessment of Bariatric Surgery (Teen-LABS) and its adult counterpart, LABS. Teens in the study were under 19 years of age at the time of surgery, and adults in the study reported having obesity by the age of 18. The Teen-LABS clinical centers had specialized experience in the surgical evaluation and management of young people with severe obesity, and both studies were funded primarily by the NIH's National Institute of Diabetes and Digestive and Kidney Diseases (NIDDK). The results were published in *The New England Journal of Medicine (NEJM)*.

"Obesity increases the risk for type 2 diabetes and cardiovascular diseases, and these conditions can be more difficult to manage in young people," said Mary Evans, Ph.D., a study author, and program director in the NIDDK Division of Digestive Diseases and Nutrition. "We found earlier bariatric surgery in carefully selected youth may have greater benefits compared to waiting until later in life."

About This Chapter: This chapter includes text excerpted from "Early Weight-Loss Surgery May Improve Type 2 Diabetes, Blood Pressure Outcomes," National Institutes of Health (NIH), May 16, 2019.

Key findings of the research include:

- Overall weight loss percentage was not different between the groups. Teens lost 26 percent of their body weight, and adults lost 29 percent at 5 years after surgery.

- Type 2 diabetes declined in both groups, but teens with type 2 diabetes before surgery were 27 percent more likely than adults to have controlled blood glucose (blood sugar) without the use of diabetes medications.

- No teens in the group needed diabetes medications after surgery, compared to 88 percent of teens before surgery. 79 percent of adults used diabetes medications before surgery, and 26 percent used diabetes medications 5 years later.

- Before surgery, 57 percent of teens and 68 percent of adults used blood pressure medications. 5 years after surgery, 11 percent of teens and 33 percent of adults used blood pressure medications.

- Among those with high blood pressure before surgery, teens were 51 percent more likely than adults to no longer have high blood pressure or take blood pressure medication.

However, teens were more likely to have increased risks in other areas, including a need for subsequent abdominal surgeries, most commonly gallbladder removal. Teens were also more likely to have low iron and vitamin D levels, potentially because teens may be less likely to take enough vitamin and mineral supplements after surgery. There was a similar death rate for both teens and adults five years after surgery, including two people from the teen group who died from overdose. There is an overall increasing trend of drug overdose deaths in the United States, and a previous LABS study found an increased risk of substance- and alcohol-use disorders after bariatric surgery in adults.

"Although there are risks associated with bariatric surgery, this study demonstrates that, for many young people, the benefits likely outweigh the risks," said Thomas Inge, M.D., Ph.D., the study's first author from Children's Hospital Colorado. "Sufficient vitamin and mineral supplementation, along with continued medical care, can help mitigate some of these risks."

These results build on earlier research related to the benefits, risks, and timing of bariatric surgery to aid in weight management. Obesity affects more than 1 in 3 adults and about 17 percent of American children and teens. Obesity increases the risk for type 2 diabetes, heart and kidney diseases, some types of cancer, and other health conditions.

"Type 2 diabetes in youth has been a growing problem without a solution, hitting young adults with serious health conditions when they should be in the prime of their lives. This study demonstrates that bariatric surgery may provide an effective treatment, though not one without risks," said NIDDK Director Dr. Griffin P. Rodgers. "We hope future research continues to shed light on the best timing and the most effective treatments for all people with weight-related conditions."

Type 2 diabetes among young people is on the rise—so is obesity. Type 2 diabetes was once thought to be a condition that developed only in older adults. Now, because obesity is common at all ages, type 2 diabetes is becoming a problem for people of all ages. This includes children and especially children of certain racial and ethnic groups, such as blacks and Hispanics. Young people with diabetes are typically overweight or obese and have a family history of diabetes. Young people who have prediabetes or diabetes are more likely to develop other disorders, including high blood pressure and high cholesterol.

(Source: "Diabetes, Heart Disease, and You," Centers for Disease Control and Prevention (CDC).)

Part Six
If You Need More Information

Chapter 51

Resources for Diabetes Information

National Institute of Diabetes and Digestive and Kidney Diseases (NIDDK)

National Diabetes Education Program (NDEP)

NIDDK Health Information Center
Toll-Free: 800-860-8747
Toll-Free TTY: 866-569-1162
Website: www.ndep.nih.gov
E-mail: healthinfo@niddk.nih.gov

National Diabetes Information Clearinghouse (NDIC)

NIDDK Health Information Center
Toll-Free: 800-860-8747
Toll-Free TTY: 866-569-1162
Website: www.diabetes.niddk.nih.gov
E-mail: healthinfo@niddk.nih.gov

National Digestive Diseases Information Clearinghouse (NDDIC)

NIDDK Health Information Center
Toll-Free: 800-860-8747
Toll-Free TTY: 866-569-1162
Website: www.digestive.niddk.nih.gov
E-mail: healthinfo@niddk.nih.gov

About This Chapter: Resources in this chapter were compiled from several sources deemed reliable; all contact information was verified and updated in June 2019.

National Kidney and Urologic Diseases Information Clearinghouse (NKUDIC)

NIDDK Health Information Center
Toll-Free: 800-860-8747
Toll-Free TTY: 866-569-1162
Website: www.kidncy.niddk.nih.gov
E-mail: healthinfo@niddk.nih.gov

National Kidney Disease Education Program (NKDEP)

NIDDK Health Information Center
Toll-Free: 800-860-8747
Toll-Free TTY: 866-569-1162
Website: www.nkdep.nih.gov
E-mail: healthinfo@niddk.nih.gov

Weight-Control Information Network (WIN)

NIDDK Health Information Center
Toll-Free: 800-860-8747
Toll-Free TTY: 866-569-1162
Website: win.niddk.nih.gov
E-mail: healthinfo@niddk.nih.gov

Diabetes Endocrinology Research Centers (DERCs)

Division of Endocrinology, Diabetes and Metabolism

Penn Medicine
Philadelphia, PA 19102
Toll-Free: 800-789-7366
Website: www.pennmedicine.org/departments-and-centers/department-of-medicine/divisions/division-of-endocrinology-diabetes-and-metabolism

Joslin Diabetes and Endocrinology Research Center (DERC)

Joslin Diabetes Center
One Joslin Pl.
Boston, MA 02215
Phone: 617-309-2400
Website: www.joslin.org/7108.html

University of Colorado Diabetes and Endocrinology Research Center (DERC)

University of Colorado School of Medicine
Anschutz Medical Campus
Aurora, CO 80045
Phone: 303-724-6836
Fax: 303-724-6838
Website: 140.226.22.38/DERC/index.htm
E-mail: Kathryn.Gray@ucdenver.edu

Diabetic Eye Disease

American Academy of Ophthalmology (AAO)

655 Beach St.
San Francisco, CA 94109
Phone: 415-561-8500
Fax: 415-561-8533
Website: www.aao.org

EyeCare America

Toll-Free: 877-887-6327
Fax: 415-561-8567
Website: www.aao.org/eyecare-america
E-mail: eyecareamerica@aao.org

Prevent Blindness

211 W. Wacker Dr.
Ste. 400
Chicago, IL 60606
Toll-Free: 800-331-2020
Website: www.preventblindness.org
E-mail: info@preventblindness.org

Diabetes-Related Bone Diseases

National Institutes of Health Osteoporosis and Related Bone Diseases—National Resource Center (NIH ORBD—NRC)

2 AMS Cir.
Bethesda, MD 20892-3676
Toll-Free: 800-624-BONE (800-624-2663)
Phone: 202-223-0344
TTY: 202-466-4315
Fax: 202-293-2356
Website: www.bones.nih.gov
E-mail: NIHBoncInfo@mail.nih. gov

Diabetes-Related Foot Problems

National Institute of Arthritis and Musculoskeletal and Skin Diseases (NIAMS)

1 AMS Cir.
Bethesda, MD 20892-3675
Toll-Free: 877-22-NIAMS (877-226-4267)
Phone: 301-495-4484
TTY: 301-565-2966
Fax: 301-718-6366
Website: www.niams.nih.gov
E-mail: NIAMSinfo@mail.nih. gov

Diabetes-Related Heart Disease

American Heart Association (AHA)

National Center
7272 Greenville Ave.
Dallas, TX 75231
Toll-Free: 800-AHA-USA-1 (800-242-8721)
Website: www.heart.org

Diabetes-Related Mouth Problems

National Institute of Dental and Craniofacial Research (NIDCR)

National Oral Health Information Clearinghouse (NOHIC)
1 NOHIC Way
Bethesda, MD 20892-3500
Toll-Free: 866-232-4528
Phone: 301-402-7364
Fax: 301-907-8830
Website: www.nidcr.nih.gov
E-mail: nohic@nidcr.nih.gov

Diabetes Research and Training Centers (DRTCs)

Albert Einstein College of Medicine Diabetes Research Center (DRC)

Jack and Pearl Resnick Campus
1300 Morris Park Ave.
Bronx, NY 10461
Phone: 718-430-2000
Website: www.einstein.yu.edu/centers/diabetes-research
E-mail: information@einstein.yu.edu

Massachusetts General Hospital (MGH) Diabetes Clinical Research Center

55 Fruit St.
Boston, MA 02114
Phone: 617-726-2000
Website: www.massgeneral.org/research/researchlab.aspx?id=1038

Michigan Diabetes Research Center (MDRC)

University of Michigan Health System (UMHS)
1000 Wall St.
Rm. 6107 Brehm Tower
Ann Arbor, MI 48105-5714
Phone: 734-763-6103
Fax: 734-647 9523
Website: diabetesresearch.med.umich.edu
E-mail: mmalec@umich.edu

The University of Chicago Diabetes Research and Training Center (DRTC)

5801 S. Ellis
Chicago, IL 60637
Website: drtc.bsd.uchicago.edu

University of Washington Diabetes Research Center (DRC)

Phone: 206-764-2688
Fax: 206-764-2693
Website: depts.washington.edu/diabetes
E-mail: drc@medicine.washington.edu

Vanderbilt Diabetes Research and Training Center (DRTC)

Vanderbilt University Medical Center (VUMC)
Phone: 615-322-7004
Website: www.vumc.org/diabetescenter/DRTC

Washington University School of Medicine (WUSM) Diabetes Research Center (DRC)

660 S. Euclid Ave.
CB 8086
St. Louis, MO 63110
Phone: 314-362-8717
Fax: 314-286-1919
Website: diabetesresearchcenter.dom.wustl.edu
E-mail: jschaff@wustl.edu

Yale Diabetes Research Center (DRC)

Yale School of Medicine (YSM)
300 Cedar St. TAC S141
New Haven, CT 06520-8020
Phone: 203-737-5071
Fax: 203-737-5558
Website: medicine.yale.edu/intmed/drc/index.aspx
E-mail: kathleen.catalano@yale.edu

Diabetic Kidney Disease

American Association of Kidney Patients (AAKP)
14440 Bruce B. Downs Blvd.
Tampa, FL 33613
Toll-Free: 800-749-AAKP (800-749-2257)
Phone: 813-636-8100
Fax: 813-636-8122
Website: aakp.org
E-mail: info@aakp.org

Urology Care Foundation
1000 Corporate Blvd.
Linthicum, MD 21090
Toll-Free: 800-828-7866
Phone: 410-689-3990
Fax: 410-689-3998
Website: www.urologyhealth.org
E-mail: auafoundation@auafoundation.org

General

Diabetes Canada (DC)
1300-522 University Ave.
Toronto, ON M5G 2R5
Toll-Free: 800-BANTING (800-226-8464)
Phone: 416-363-3373
Website: www.diabetes.ca
E-mail: info@diabetes.ca

Diabetes Center of Excellence (DCOE)
University of Massachusetts Medical School (UMMS)
368 Plantation St.
Albert Sherman Center AS7.2046
Worcester, MA 01605
Phone: 508-455-3654
Website: www.umassmed.edu/dcoe
E-mail: lisa.hubacz@umassmed.edu

Diabetes Teaching Center

University of California, San Francisco (UCSF)
400 Parnassus Ave.
Ste. A-550
San Francisco, CA 94143
Toll-Free: 888-689-UCSF (888-689-8273)
Phone: 415-353-2266
Fax: 415-353-2337
Website: www.ucsfhealth.org/clinics/diabetes_teaching_center/?refid=glocalsearch

Indiana University Diabetes Translational Research Program

Center for Diabetes and Metabolic Diseases (CDMD)
Van Nuys Medical Science Bldg. 635 Barnhill Dr.
Ste. 2031A
Indianapolis, IN 46202
Website: medicine.iu.edu/research/centers-institutes/diabetes-metabolic-diseases/research/translational/

Johns Hopkins Diabetes Center

601 N. Caroline St.
Ste. 2008
Baltimore, MD 21287
Phone: 410-955-9270
TTY: 410-955-6217
Website: www.hopkinsmedicine.org/diabetes/mission.html

Joslin Diabetes Center

One Joslin Pl.
Boston, MA 02215
Phone: 617-309-2400
Website: www.joslin.org

Office of Minority Health Resource Center (OMHRC)

Toll-Free: 800-444-6472
Phone: 240-453-2882
TDD: 301-251-1432
Fax: 301-251-2160
Website: www.minorityhealth.hhs.gov
E-mail: info@minorityhealth.hhs.gov

Juvenile Diabetes

Barbara Davis Center for Childhood Diabetes (BDC)
1775 Aurora Ct.
Aurora, CO 80045
Phone: 303-724-2323
Fax: 303-724-6839
Website: www.barbaradaviscenter.org

Children with Diabetes, Inc. (CWD)
Website: childrenwithdiabetes.com

The Nemours Foundation/KidsHealth®
10140 Centurion Pkwy N.
Jacksonville, FL 32256
Phone: 904-697-4100
Website: www.nemours.org

Other Resources at the National Institutes of Health (NIH)

National Center for Complementary and Integrative Health (NCCIH)
Clearinghouse
9000 Rockville Pike
Bethesda, MD 20892
Toll-Free: 888-644-6226
Toll-Free TTY: 866-464-3615
Website: nccih.nih.gov
E-mail: info@nccih.nih.gov

National Eye Institute (NEI)
Office of Science Communications, Public Liaison, and Education (OSCPLE)
31 Center Dr. MSC 2510
Bethesda, MD 20892-2510
Phone: 301-496-5248
Website: www.nei.nih.gov
E-mail: 2020@nei.nih.gov

National Heart, Lung, and Blood Institute (NHLBI)
Health Information Center
P.O. Box 30105
Bethesda, MD 20824-0105
Phone: 301-592-8573
Website: www.nhlbi.nih.gov
E-mail: nhlbiinfo@nhlbi.nih.gov

National Institute of Arthritis and Musculoskeletal and Skin Diseases (NIAMS)
1 AMS Cir.
Bethesda, MD 20892-3675
Toll-Free: 877-22-NIAMS (877-226-4267)
Phone: 301-495-4484
TTY: 301-565-2966
Fax: 301-718-6366
Website: www.niams.nih.gov
E-mail: NIAMSinfo@mail.nih. gov

National Institute of Dental and Craniofacial Research (NIDCR)
National Oral Health Information Clearinghouse (NOHIC)
1 NOHIC Way
Bethesda, MD 20892-3500
Toll-Free: 866-232-4528
Phone: 301-402-7364
Fax: 301-907-8830
Website: www.nidcr.nih.gov
E-mail: nohic@nidcr.nih.gov

National Institute on Aging (NIA)
Information Center
31 Center Dr. MSC 2292
Bldg. 31 Rm. 5C27
Bethesda, MD 20892
Toll-Free: 800-222-2225
Toll-Free TTY: 800-222-4225
Website: www.nia.nih.gov
E-mail: niaic@nia.nih.gov

Other Resources at the U.S. Department of Health and Human Services (HHS)

Diabetes Care

U.S. Department of Veterans Affairs (VA)
Toll-Free: 844-MyVA311 (844-698-2311)
TTY: 711-698-2311
Website: www.va.gov/QUALITYOFCARE/improving/Diabetes_research.asp

Division of Diabetes Translation

Centers for Disease Control and Prevention (CDC)
1600 Clifton Rd.
Atlanta, GA 30329-4027
Toll-Free: 800-CDC-INFO (800-232-4636)
Toll-Free TTY: 888-232-6348
Website: www.cdc.gov/diabetes

Office of Minority Health Resource Center (OMHRC)

U.S. Department of Health and Human Services (HHS)
Toll-Free: 800-444-6472
TDD: 301-251-1432
Fax: 301-251-2160
Website: www.minorityhealth.hhs.gov
E-mail: info@minorityhealth.hhs.gov

Professional and Consumer Healthcare Associations

Academy of Nutrition and Dietetics

120 S. Riverside Plaza
Ste. 2190
Chicago, IL 60606-6995
Toll-Free: 800-877-1600
Phone: 312-899-0040
Website: www.eatright.org

American Association of Clinical Endocrinologists (AACE)

245 Riverside Ave.
Ste. 200
Jacksonville, FL 32202
Phone: 904-353-7878
Fax: 240-547-0026
Website: www.aace.com

American Association of Diabetes Educators (AADE)

200 W. Madison St.
Ste. 800
Chicago, IL 60606
Toll-Free: 800-338-3633
Website: www.diabeteseducator.org

American Diabetes Association (ADA)

2451 Crystal Dr.
Ste. 900
Arlington, VA 22202
Toll-Free: 800-DIABETES (800-342-2383)
Website: www.diabetes.org
E-mail: askada@diabetes.org

American Podiatric Medical Association (APMA)

9312 Old Georgetown Rd.
Bethesda, MD 20814-1621
Phone: 301-581-9200
Website: www.apma.org

Diabetes Action Research and Education Foundation (Diabetes Action)

P.O. Box 34635
Bethesda, MD 20827
Phone: 202-333-4520
Fax: 202-558-5240
Website: diabetesaction.org
E-mail: info@diabetesaction.org

Endocrine Society

2055 L. St. N.W.
Ste. 600
Washington, DC 20036
Toll-Free: 888-363-6274
Phone: 202-971-3636
Fax: 202-736-9705
Website: www.endocrine.org
E-mail: info@endocrine.org

Juvenile Diabetes Research Foundation (JDRF)

26 Bdwy.
14th Fl.
New York, NY 10004
Toll-Free: 800-533-CURE (800-533-2873)
Fax: 212-785-9595
Website: www.jdrf.org
E-mail: info@jdrf.org

National Certification Board For Diabetes Educators (NCBDE)

330 E. Algonquin Rd.
Ste. 4
Arlington Heights, IL 60005
Toll-Free: 877-239-3233
Phone: 847-228-9795
Fax: 847-228-8469
Website: www.ncbde.org
E-mail: info@ncbde.org

National Glycohemoglobin Standardization Program (NGSP)

Website: www.ngsp.org
E-mail: ngsp@missouri.edu

National Kidney Foundation (NKF)

30 E. 33rd St.
New York, NY 10016
Toll-Free: 800-622-9010
Fax: 212-689-9261
Website: www.kidney.org
E-mail: info@kidney.org

Pedorthic Footcare Association (PFA)

P.O. Box 72184
Albany, GA 31708-2184
Toll-Free: 888-563-0945
Phone: 229-389-3440
Website: www.pedorthics.org
E-mail: info@pedorthics.org

Urology Care Foundation

1000 Corporate Boulevard
Linthicum, MD 21090
Toll-Free: 800-828-7866
Phone: 410-689-3990
Fax: 410-689-3998
Website: www.urologyhealth.org
E-mail: auafoundation@auafoundation.org

Chapter 52

Finding Diabetes-Friendly Recipes

Healthy Food for Diabetics

For people with diabetes, knowing what to serve and eat for family dinners can be tough. Eating healthy is key to all sorts of health benefits such as lowering blood pressure and stronger bones. However, it is important for people with diabetes since eating healthy foods can help keep their blood sugar within a healthy target range. This is a critical part of managing diabetes since controlling your blood sugar can prevent the complications of diabetes.

Diabetics' Dinner Dilemma

Whether you have diabetes or someone you know does, you can prepare a group meal that is healthy and tastes great. While reviewing recipes measure each meal's carbohydrates since they are the main nutrient that affects blood sugar. People with diabetes can balance their total carbohydrates throughout the day by eating appropriate portion sizes for meals and snacks.

What to Include and Avoid

Look for recipes that are low in saturated fats, trans fats, cholesterol, salt (sodium), and added sugars. Try meals that include fiber-rich foods because they can delay the absorption

About This Chapter: Text under the heading "Healthy Food for Diabetics" is excerpted from "Recipes for a Diabetic-Friendly Meal," U.S. Department of Veterans Affairs (VA), October 19, 2018; Text under the heading "Some Recipes for You to Try" is excerpted from "Tasty Recipes," Centers for Disease Control and Prevention (CDC), March 2011. Reviewed June 2019.

of sugar. This can help someone with diabetes control their blood sugar. When choosing from these food groups you should:

- Fruits

- Include: Oranges, melons, berries, apples, and bananas

- Avoid: Grapes, cherries, and pineapples

- Vegetables

- Include: Broccoli, carrots, greens, peppers, and tomatoes

- Avoid: Potatoes, corn, and green peas

- Protein

- Include: Lean meat (chicken or turkey without the skin), fish, eggs, nuts and peanuts, dried beans and certain peas, and meat substitutes like tofu

- Avoid: Fried meat, pork bacon, cut lunch meats

- Whole grains

- Include: Wheat, rice, oats, cornmeal, barley, and quinoa

- Avoid: White bread, pasta, tortillas, and sugary cereal

- Dairy

- Include: Low-fat or nonfat milk, cheese, and yogurt

- Avoid: Whole milk, regular cheese, and yogurt

Delicious Meals Everyone Can Enjoy

The U.S. Department of Veterans Affairs (VA) offers a variety of delicious, healthy recipes in the *Yummy Benefits Cookbook* and *Yummy Benefits Cookbook II*. These meals are packed with healthy ingredients but don't lack flavor. A few diabetes-friendly recipes you should try:

- Garlic citrus fish—a protein-packed recipe using cod or tilapia. Include garlic to provide extra flavor, but also help maintain blood sugar levels as well as reduce your risk of heart disease.

- Black bean turkey chili—a delicious and healthy take on traditional chili. This recipe combines lean turkey meat with black beans to provide a meal rich in both protein and fiber. Opting for low sodium diced tomatoes in this dish reduces your risk of heart disease, a common diabetes complication.

- Colorful winter quinoa salad—a seasonal meat-free option that uses leafy greens as a tasty way to manage blood sugar levels. Using red wine vinegar in your dressing allows you to cut calories without leaving your salad bland.

Some Recipes for You to Try

Diabetic exchanges are calculated based on the American Diabetes Association Exchange System. Percent Daily Values are based on a 2,000 calorie diet.

Spanish Omelet

This tasty dish provides a healthy array of vegetables and can be used for breakfast, brunch, or any meal. Serve with fresh fruit salad and a whole grain dinner roll.

Nutrition Facts

- Serving Size: ⅕ of omelet

Amount per Serving

- Calories 260

- Calories from fat 90

% Daily Value (DV)

- Total fat 10 g, 15%

- Saturated fat 3.5 g, 18%

- Trans fat 0 g

- Cholesterol 135 mg, 45%

- Sodium 240 mg, 10%

- Total carbohydrate 30 g, 10%

- Dietary fiber 3 g, 12%

- Sugars 3 g

- Protein 16 g

- Vitamin A 8%

- Vitamin C 60%

- Calcium 15%

- Iron 8%

Ingredients

- 5 small potatoes, peeled and sliced

- vegetable cooking spray

- ½ medium onion, minced

- 1 small zucchini, sliced

- 1½ cups green/red peppers, sliced thin

- 5 medium mushrooms, sliced

- 3 whole eggs, beaten

- 5 egg whites, beaten

- pepper and garlic salt with herbs, to taste

- 3 ounces shredded part-skim mozzarella cheese

- 1 tablespoon low-fat parmesan cheese

Directions

- Preheat oven to 375°F.

- Cook potatoes in boiling water until tender.

- In a nonstick pan, add vegetable spray and warm at medium heat.

- Add onion and sauté until brown. Add vegetables and sauté until tender but not brown.

- In a medium mixing bowl, slightly beat eggs and egg whites, pepper, garlic salt, and low-fat mozzarella cheese. Stir egg-cheese mixture into the cooked vegetables.

- In a 10-inch pie pan or ovenproof skillet, add vegetable spray and transfer potatoes and egg mixture to pan. Sprinkle with low-fat parmesan cheese and bake until firm and brown on top, about 20 to 30 minutes.

- Remove omelet from oven, cool for 10 minutes, and cut into five pieces.

Exchanges

- Meat 2

- Bread 2

- Vegetable ⅔

- Fat 2

Beef or Turkey Stew

This dish goes nicely with a green leaf lettuce and cucumber salad and a dinner roll. Plantains or corn can be used in place of the potatoes.

Nutrition Facts

- Serving Size: 1½ cup

Amount per Serving

- Calories: 320

- Calories from fat: 60

% Daily Value (DV)

- Total fat 7g, 11%

- Saturated fat 1.5 g, 8%

- Trans fat 0 g

- Cholesterol 40 mg, 13%

- Sodium 520 mg, 22%

- Total carbohydrate 41 g, 14%

- Dietary fiber 8 g, 32%

- Sugars 9 g
- Protein 24 g
- Vitamin A 340%
- Vitamin C 80%
- Calcium 6%
- Iron 15%

Ingredients

- 1 pound lean beef or turkey breast, cut into cubes
- 2 tbsp. whole wheat flour
- ¼ tsp. salt (optional)
- ¼ tsp. pepper
- ¼ tsp. cumin
- 1½ Tbsp. olive oil
- 2 cloves garlic, minced
- 2 medium onions, sliced
- 2 stalks celery, sliced
- 1 medium red/green bell pepper, sliced
- 1 medium tomato, finely minced
- 5 cups beef or turkey broth, fat removed
- 5 small potatoes, peeled and cubed
- 12 small carrots, cut into large chunks
- 1¼ cups green peas

Directions

- Preheat oven to 375°F.
- Mix the whole wheat flour with salt, pepper, and cumin. Roll the beef or turkey cubes in the mixture. Shake off excess flour.

- In a large skillet, heat olive oil over medium-high heat. Add beef or turkey cubes and sauté until nicely brown, about 7 to 10 minutes.

- Place beef or turkey in an ovenproof casserole dish.

- Add minced garlic, onions, celery, and peppers to skillet and cook until vegetables are tender, about five minutes.

- Stir in tomato and broth. Bring to a boil and pour over turkey or beef in casserole dish. Cover dish tightly and bake for one hour at 375°F.

- Remove from oven and stir in potatoes, carrots, and peas. Bake for another 20 to 25 minutes or until tender.

Exchanges

- Lean meat 3
- Vegetable 2½
- Bread 2⅔
- Fat 1

Two Cheese Pizza

Serve your pizza with fresh fruit and a mixed green salad garnished with red beans to balance your meal.

Nutrition Facts

- Serving Size: 2 slices (¼ of pie)

Amount per Serving

- Calories: 420
- Calories from fat: 170

% Daily Value (DV)

- Total fat 19 g, 29%
- Saturated fat 7 g, 35%
- Trans fat 0 g

- Cholesterol 25 mg, 8%

- Sodium 580 mg, 24%

- Total carbohydrate 44 g, 15%

- Dietary fiber 3 g, 12%

- Sugars 5 g

- Protein 20 g

- Vitamin A 30%

- Vitamin C 90%

- Calcium 40%

- Iron 15%

Ingredients

- 2 Tbsp. whole wheat flour

- 1 can (10 ounces) refrigerated pizza crust

- Vegetable cooking spray

- 2 Tbsp. olive oil

- ½ cup low-fat ricotta cheese

- ½ tsp. dried basil

- 1 small onion, minced

- 2 cloves garlic, minced

- ¼ tsp. salt (optional)

- 4 ounces shredded part-skim mozzarella cheese

- 2 cups mushrooms, chopped

- 1 large red pepper, cut into strips

Directions

- Preheat oven to 425°F.

- Spread whole wheat flour over working surface. Roll out dough with rolling pin to desired crust thickness.

- Coat cookie sheet with vegetable cooking spray. Transfer pizza crust to cookie sheet. Brush olive oil over crust.

- Mix low-fat ricotta cheese with dried basil, onion, garlic, and salt. Spread this mixture over crust.

- Sprinkle crust with part-skim mozzarella cheese. Top cheese with mushrooms and red pepper.

- Bake at 425°F for 13 to 15 minutes or until cheese melts and crust is deep golden brown.

- Cut into 8 slices.

Exchanges

- Meat 2½

- Bread 3

- Vegetable 1

- Fat 3¾

Rice with Chicken, Spanish Style

This is a good way to get vegetables into the meal plan. Serve with a mixed green salad and some whole wheat bread.

Nutrition Facts

- Serving Size: 1½ cup

Amount per Serving

- Calories 400

- Calories from fat 60

% Daily Value (DV)

- Total fat 7 g, 11%

- Saturated fat 1.5 g, 8%

- Trans fat 0 g

- Cholesterol 85 mg, 28%

- Sodium 530 mg, 22%

- Total carbohydrate 46 g, 15%

- Dietary fiber 3 g, 12%

- Sugars 5 g

- Protein 37 g

- Vitamin A 30%

- Vitamin C 70%

- Calcium 4%

- Iron 20%

Ingredients

- 2 Tbsp. olive oil

- 2 medium onions, chopped

- 6 cloves garlic, minced

- 2 stalks celery, diced

- 2 medium red/green peppers, cut into strips

- 1 cup mushrooms, chopped

- 2 cups uncooked whole grain rice

- 3 pounds boneless chicken breast, cut into bite-sized pieces, skin removed

- 1½ tsp. salt (optional)

- 2½ cups low-fat chicken broth

- Saffron or Sazón™ for color

- 3 medium tomatoes, chopped

- 1 cup frozen peas

- 1 cup frozen corn
- 1 cup frozen green beans

Olives or capers for garnish (optional)

Directions

- Heat olive oil over medium heat in a nonstick pot. Add onion, garlic, celery, red/green pepper, and mushrooms. Cook over medium heat, stirring often, for three minutes or until tender.
- Add whole grain rice and sauté for two to three minutes, stirring constantly to mix all ingredients.
- Add chicken, salt, chicken broth, water, Saffron/Sazón™, and tomatoes. Bring water to a boil.
- Reduce heat to medium-low, cover, and let the casserole simmer until water is absorbed and rice is tender, about 20 minutes.
- Stir in peas, corn, and beans and cook for 8 to 10 minutes. When everything is hot, the casserole is ready to serve. Garnish with olives or capers, if desired.

Exchanges

- Meat 5⅓
- Bread 3
- Vegetable 1
- Fat 1⅓

Pozole

Only a small amount of oil is needed to sauté meat.

Nutrition Facts

- Serving Size: 1 cup

Amount per Serving

- Calories: 220

- Calories from fat: 70

% Daily Value (DV)

- Total fat 7 g, 11%

- Saturated fat 2 g, 10%

- Trans fat 0 g

- Cholesterol 70 mg, 23%

- Sodium 390 mg, 16%

- Total carbohydrate 17 g, 6%

- Dietary fiber 3 g, 12%

- Sugars 5 g

- Protein 21 g

- Vitamin A 4%

- Vitamin C 10%

- Calcium 4%

- Iron 15%

Ingredients

- 2 pounds lean beef, cubed

- 1 Tbsp. olive oil

- 1 large onion, chopped

- 1 clove garlic, finely chopped

- ¼ tsp. salt

- ⅛ tsp. pepper

- ¼ cup fresh cilantro, chopped

- 1 can (15 ounces) stewed tomatoes

- 2 ounces tomato paste

- 1 can (1 pound 13 ounces) hominy

Directions

- In a large pot, heat olive oil. Add beef and sauté. Only a small amount of oil is needed to sauté meat.
- Add onion, garlic, salt, pepper, cilantro, and enough water to cover meat. Stir to mix ingredients evenly. Cover pot and cook over low heat until meat is tender.
- Add tomatoes and tomato paste. Continue cooking for about 20 minutes.
- Add hominy and continue cooking another 15 minutes, stirring occasionally. If too thick, add water for desired consistency.

Option: Skinless, boneless chicken breasts can be used instead of beef cubes.

Exchanges

- Meat 3
- Bread 1
- Vegetable ½
- Fat 1⅓

Avocado Tacos

These fresh tasting tacos are great for a light meal.

Nutrition Facts

- Serving Size: 1 taco

Amount per Serving

- Calories: 270
- Calories from fat: 80

% Daily Value (DV)

- Total fat 8 g, 12%
- Saturated fat 2 g, 10%
- Trans fat 0 g

- Cholesterol 0 mg, 0%
- Sodium 460 mg, 19%
- Total carbohydrate 43 g, 14%
- Dietary fiber 5 g, 20%
- Sugars 4 g
- Protein 7 g
- Vitamin A 25%
- Vitamin C 100%
- Calcium 10%
- Iron 15%

Ingredients

- 1 medium onion, cut into thin strips
- 2 large green peppers, cut into thin strips
- 2 large red peppers, cut into thin strips
- 1 cup fresh cilantro, finely chopped
- 1 ripe avocado, peeled and seeded, cut into 12 slices
- 1½ cups fresh tomato salsa (see ingredients below)
- 12 flour tortillas
- Vegetable cooking spray

Fresh Tomato Salsa Ingredients

- 1 cup tomatoes, diced
- ⅓ cup onions, diced
- ½ clove garlic, minced
- 2 tsp. cilantro
- ⅓ tsp. jalapeño peppers, chopped
- ½ tsp. lime juice
- Pinch of cumin

Directions

- Mix together all salsa ingredients and refrigerate in advance.

- Coat skillet with vegetable spray.

- Lightly sauté onion and green and red peppers.

- Warm tortillas in oven and fill with peppers, onions, avocado, and salsa. Fold tortillas and serve. Top with cilantro.

Exchanges

- Bread 3

- Vegetable 1

- Fat 1½

Tropical Fruits Fantasia

The tropics offer a great variety of fruits that will make this delicious and colorful recipe stand out; it will also make your mouth water even before tasting it.

Nutrition Facts

- Serving Size: ½ cup

Amount per Serving

- Calories: 170

- Calories from fat: 5

% Daily Value (DV)

- Total fat 0.5 g, 1%

- Saturated fat 0 g, 0%

- Trans fat 0 g

- Cholesterol 0 mg, 0%

- Sodium 40 mg, 2%

- Total carbohydrate 41 g, 14%

- Dietary fiber 5 g, 20%
- Sugars 30 g
- Protein 4 g
- Vitamin A 50%
- Vitamin C 230%
- Calcium 15%
- Iron 2%

Ingredients

- 8 ounces fat-free, sugar-free orange yogurt
- 5 medium strawberries, cut into halves
- 3 ounces honeydew melon, cut into slices (or ½ cup cut into cubes)
- 3 ounces cantaloupe melon, cut into slices (or ½ cup cut into cubes)
- 1 mango, peeled and seeded, cut into cubes
- 1 papaya, peeled and seeded, cut into cubes
- 3 ounces watermelon, seeded and cut into slices (or ½ cup cut into cubes)
- 2 oranges, seeded and cut into slices
- ½ cup unsweetened orange juice

Directions

- Add yogurt and all fruits to a bowl and carefully mix together
- Pour orange juice over fruit mixture.
- Mix well and serve ½ cup as your dessert.

Exchanges

- Fruit 2¾
- Milk ⅓

Index

Index

Page numbers that appear in *Italics* refer to tables or illustrations. Page numbers that have a small 'n' after the page number refer to citation information shown as Notes. Page numbers that appear in **Bold** refer to information contained in boxes within the chapters.

A

Academy of Nutrition and Dietetics, contact 305
acanthosis nigricans (AN)
    insulin resistance and prediabetes 30
    overview 191–2
"Acanthosis Nigricans" (GARD) 191n
acarbose, hypoglycemia 120
adult-onset diabetes *see* type 2 diabetes
aerobic exercise, type 2 diabetes 50
aflibercept, diabetic eye disease 157
African Americans
    acanthosis nigricans (AN) **192**
    diabetic eye disease 155
    diabetic kidney disease 162
    type 2 diabetes **43**
Alaska Natives
    diabetes statistics 5
    diabetic eye disease 155
    type 2 diabetes **43**
Albert Einstein College of Medicine Diabetes Research Center (DRC), contact 299
alcohol use, diabetic neuropathy **149**
alpha-lipoic acid, described 273
"Alternative Devices for Taking Insulin" (NIDDK) 111n
American Academy of Ophthalmology (AAO), contact 297

American Association of Clinical Endocrinologists (AACE), contact 306
American Association of Diabetes Educators (AADE), contact 306
American Association of Kidney Patients (AAKP), contact 301
American Diabetes Association (ADA), contact 306
American Heart Association (AHA), contact 298
American Indians
    diabetes statistics 7
    diabetic eye disease 155
    diabetic kidney disease 162
    gestational diabetes **53**
    insulin resistance and prediabetes 29
    type 2 diabetes 43
American Podiatric Medical Association (APMA), contact 306
amputations
    carbohydrate counting 267
    diabetes complications 5
    hyperglycemia 122
amyloidosis, gastroparesis 168
angina, heart attack 144
angiotensin-converting-enzyme (ACE) inhibitors, diabetic kidney disease 163
angiotensin II receptor blockers (ARBs), diabetic kidney disease 163

anti-vascular endothelial growth factor (anti-VEGF) medicines, diabetic eye disease 157
antidepressants, defined 170
antiemetics, defined 170
anxiety
 description 203
 diabetic neuropathy 150
A1C test *see* hemoglobin A1C test
ARBs *see* angiotensin II receptor blockers
artificial pancreas
 diabetes medicines **107**
 insulin delivery devices 113
 type 1 diabetes 37
athlete's foot, foot problems 184
autoimmune factors, diabetic neuropathy **149**
autosomal dominant, monogenic diabetes 61
autosomal recessive, monogenic diabetes 61

B

Barbara Davis Center for Childhood Diabetes (BDC), contact 303
bariatric surgery, diabetes medicines **107**
behavioral intervention, diabetes care team 69
belly fat, heart disease 141
bevacizumab, anti-VEGF medicine 157
"Beware of Illegally Marketed Diabetes Treatments" (FDA) 125n
bezoars, gastroparesis 168
birth control, described 54
blindness
 carbohydrate counting 267
 diabetes complications 5
 diabetes management 211
 diabetic eye disease 153
 hyperglycemia 122
 smoking 240
 vision problems 136
blisters, foot problems 134
blood clot
 high blood pressure 52
 metabolic syndrome 24
 omega-3 fatty acid supplements 275
 traveling 225
blood glucose levels
 carbohydrate counting 266
 continuous glucose monitoring (CGM) 94
 diabetes management 211
 diabetes medicines 105

blood glucose levels, *continued*
 diabetic neuropathy 148
 gastroparesis 170
 hyperglycemia 121
 insulin delivery devices 111
 insulin resistance 27
 managing diabetes **75**
 nerve damage 133
 pregnancy 232
 sexual problems 196
 type 1 diabetes 36
blood glucose monitoring, overview 89–96
"Blood Glucose Monitoring Devices" (FDA) 89n
blood pressure
 diabetes care team 69
 diabetes medicines 106
 diabetic kidney disease 163
 diabetic neuropathy 150
 gestational diabetes 52
 heart disease 131
 managing diabetes **75**
 metabolic syndrome 18
 physical activity **276**
 pregnancy **232**
 sexual and bladder problems 194
 smoking 241
 type 1 diabetes 39
 type 2 diabetes 43
blood sugar *see* blood glucose levels
blood sugar meter, diabetes management 212
blood sugar monitor
 managing diabetes 237
 traveling 224
 type 1 diabetes 49
blood tests
 glucose in urine test 97
 insulin resistance and prediabetes 30
 maturity-onset diabetes 59
 metabolic syndrome 21
 type 2 diabetes 42
 see also blood glucose monitoring; fingerstick test
blood vessel disease, carbohydrate counting 267
blood vessels
 A1C test 78
 diabetic eye disease 154
 diabetic kidney disease 162
 heart disease 131
 pregnancy 233
 sexual and bladder problems 193
 smoking 140

BMI *see* body mass index
body fat, heart disease **140**
body mass index (BMI), insulin resistance and prediabetes 30
breakfast, meal plans and diabetes **261**

C

calluses, foot problems 134
calories
    diabetes myths 64
    gastroparesis 169
    obesity 141
    type 2 diabetes 43
    weight-loss planning 261
candidiasis, tabulated *177*
carbohydrate counting
    meal plan methods 262
    overview 265–71
"Carbohydrate Counting and Diabetes" (NIDDK) 265n
cardiovascular disease (CVD)
    diabetes care team 69
    diabetes medicines 109
    metabolic syndrome **24**
carpal tunnel syndrome (CTS), diabetic neuropathy **149**
cataracts, diabetic eye disease 153
Centers for Disease Control and Prevention (CDC)
    publications
        coping with diabetes distress 207n
        diabetes and mental health 203n
        diabetes and women 51n
        diabetes management team 69n
        diabetes myths 63n
        diabetes quick facts 3n
        diabetes risks 9n
        diabetes statistics 3n
        family health history and diabetes 9n
        friends, family, and diabetes 243n
        gestational diabetes and pregnancy 51n
        healthy food choices for diabetes 253n
        healthy weight 285n
        ketones in urine test 101n
        managing diabetes in the heat 235n
        physical activity and diabetes 279n
        prevent diabetes-related complications 131n
        smoking and diabetes 239n
        traveling with diabetes 223n

cereals, carbohydrate counting 266
CGM *see* continuous glucose monitor
Charcot's foot, foot problems 184
chest pain
    hyperglycemia 123
    metabolic syndrome 17
Children with Diabetes, Inc. (CWD), website address 303
cholesterol levels
    carbohydrate counting 265
    diabetic neuropathy 150
    heart disease 132
    metabolic syndrome 23
    smoking 142
chromium, dietary supplements 274
chronic kidney disease (CKD) *see* kidney disease
CKD *see* chronic kidney disease
continuous glucose monitoring (CGM)
    artificial pancreas 113
    overview 94–6
    see also blood glucose monitoring
"Continuous Glucose Monitoring" (NIDDK) 89n
CTS *see* carpal tunnel syndrome
Cushing syndrome, insulin resistance 29
CVD *see* cardiovascular disease
cystic fibrosis, diabetes 4
cystitis, bladder infections 198

D

dairy products, carbohydrates 266
damaged nerves
    diabetes 133
    smoking 240
"Definition and Facts for Gastroparesis" (NIDDK) 167n
dehydration
    diabetic ketoacidosis 122
    gastroparesis 168
    heat 235
    neonatal diabetes mellitus 58
    physical activity 282
delayed gastric emptying
    digestive problems 134
    see also gastroparesis
dental cleaning, oral health 136
dentist
    oral health 136
    plaque 176

dentures
    oral health 181
    tabulated *136*
depression
    diabetes 203
    diabetic neuropathy 150
    mental health 137
    metabolic syndrome 20
    type 1 diabetes 39
    women **53**
diabetes
    blood glucose 89
    blood sugar 83
    carbohydrate counting 265
    children 13
    distress 207
    driving 219
    eyes 153
    foot and skin problems 183
    health concerns 131
    healthcare team 69
    healthy eating 249
    heart disease 139
    heat 235
    hypoglycemia 115
    insulin delivery 111
    insulin resistance 27
    kidneys 161
    management 75
    meal plans 259
    medicines 105
    mental health 203
    monogenic forms 57
    mouth 175
    myths 63
    physical activities 279
    school 211
    sexual problems 193
    smoking 239
    statistics 3
    treatment fraud 125
    urine test 97
    weight loss 289
    women 51
Diabetes Action Research and Education
   Foundation(Diabetes Action), contact 306
"Diabetes and Dietary Supplements" (NCCIH) 273n
"Diabetes and Foot Problems" (NIDDK) 183n
"Diabetes and Mental Health" (CDC) 203n

"Diabetes and Women" (CDC) 51n
Diabetes Canada (DC), contact 301
Diabetes Care, contact 305
Diabetes Center of Excellence (DCOE), contact 301
Diabetes Control and Complications Trial (DCCT),
   blood glucose monitoring 90
"Diabetes Diet, Eating, and Physical Activity"
   (NIDDK) 259n
diabetes diet, healthy eating 249
diabetes distress
    described 205
    mental health 137
"Diabetes—Eat Well" (CDC) 253n
diabetes educators
    carbohydrates *267*
    diabetes distress 206
    diabetes management 76
    healthy eating 257
    traveling 225
diabetes-friendly diet *see* mealtime; meal plan
"Diabetes—Get Active!" (CDC) 279n
"Diabetes, Gum Disease and Other Dental Problems"
   (NIDDK) 175n
"Diabetes, Heart Disease, and Stroke"
   (NIDDK) 139n
"Diabetes in Children and Teens" (NIH) 13n
diabetes medications
    blood glucose control 211
    blood sugar 53
    weight loss 290
diabetes mellitus
    acanthosis nigricans (AN) 191
    type 1 diabetes **34**
diabetes myths, overview 63–5
"Diabetes Myths" (CDC) 63n
diabetes pills *see* medications
Diabetes Prevention Program (DPP)
    insulin resistance 31
    type 2 diabetes 44
"Diabetes Quick Facts" (CDC) 3n
"Diabetes Report Card 2017" (CDC) 3n
"Diabetes, Sexual, and Bladder Problems"
   (NIDDK) 193n
diabetes supplies
    ketones test **103**
    Medicare 82
    traveling 224
Diabetes Teaching Center, contact 302
"Diabetic Eye Disease" (NIDDK) 153n

diabetic ketoacidosis (DKA)
    hyperglycemia 122
    ketones 101
    neonatal diabetes mellitus 58
    type 1 diabetes 34
diabetic kidney disease
    defined 132
    overview 161–5
"Diabetic Kidney Disease" (NIDDK) 161n
diabetic macular edema, eye disease 153
diabetic nephropathy, kidneys 132
diabetic neuropathy
    dietary supplements 273
    foot and skin 183
    overview 147–51
    sexual problems 193
diabetic retinopathy see retinopathy
dialysis, kidney disease 132
dietary supplements
    overview 273–8
    pediatric patients 110
    unapproved drugs 126
dietitian, diabetes care 71
diets
    carbohydrate 267
    chronic kidney disease (CKD) 256
    glucose 89
    weight management 285
digestion
    diabetic neuropathy 147
    gastroparesis 167
    nerve damage 134
    non-starchy vegetables 249
    pediatric patients 109
digestive system
    carbohydrates 266
    hypoglycemia 117
dilated eye exam
    cardiovascular health 72
    diabetic eye disease 153
    vision 136
diuretics, heat 235
Division of Diabetes Translation, contact 305
Division of Endocrinology, Diabetes and Metabolism, contact 296
DKA see diabetic ketoacidosis
domperidone, blood glucose levels 170
double diabetes, overview 47–50
"Double Diabetes" (Omnigraphics) 47n

"Driving When You Have Diabetes" (NHTSA) 219n

E

"Early Weight-Loss Surgery May Improve Type 2 Diabetes, Blood Pressure Outcomes" (NIH) 289n
"Eating, Diet, and Nutrition for Gastroparesis" (NIDDK) 167n
eating disorders, gastroparesis 168
ECG see electrocardiogram
ED see erectile dysfunction
edema, laser treatment 157
electrocardiogram (ECG), double diabetes 49
emergencies
    medical alert jewelry 216
    summer checklist **236**
Endocrine Society, contact 307
environmental factors, monogenic forms 57
erectile dysfunction (ED)
    sexual problems 193
    type 2 diabetes 48
erythromycin, gastroparesis 170
exercises
    blood sugar 85
    children 14
    stress 205
    type 2 diabetes 50
    weight management 286
    see also physical activity
EyeCare America, contact 297
eyes
    A1C test 78
    diabetic eye disease 153
    diabetic neuropathy 148
    driving 219
    maturity-onset diabetes 59
    metabolic syndrome 24
    see also retinopathy; vision problems

F

fad diets, healthy weight 285
family health history, diabetes 11
"Family Health History and Diabetes" (CDC) 9n
family history
    diabetic kidney disease 162
    heart disease 141
    insulin resistance 29

family history, *continued*
    maturity-onset diabetes 59
    necrobiosis lipoidica 192
    prediabetes **11**
    type 2 diabetes 41
fast-acting carbs, backpack checklist **212**
fasting plasma glucose (FPG)
    double diabetes 48
    insulin resistance 31
fatigue
    glucose 98
    hyperglycemia 121
    metabolic syndrome 19
    type 1 diabetes 34
FDA *see* U.S. Food and Drug Administration
"FDA Approves New Treatment for Pediatric
    Patients with Type 2 Diabetes" (FDA) 105n
feet
    A1C test 78
    diabetes 42, 183
    diabetic neuropathy 149
    driving 219
    metabolic syndrome 24
    nerve damage 133
    physical activity 283
    smoking 240
fluids
    diabetes 282
    hyperglycemia **123**
    skin 189
focal neuropathies, defined 148
Food and Drug Administration *see* U.S. Food and
    Drug Administration
food portions, healthy eating 249
foot ulcers, diabetes 183
"4 Steps to Manage Your Diabetes for Life"
    (NIDDK) 75n
FPG *see* fasting plasma glucose
fraud, diabetes treatment 125
"Friends, Family, and Diabetes" (CDC) 243n

G

gallbladder
    pediatric patients 109
    weight-loss surgery 290
gallstones
    healthy weight **285**
    metabolic syndrome 19

gangrene, diabetes 180
gastric electrical stimulation (GES), gastroparesis 172
gastroparesis
    diabetes 134
    overview 167–73
gastrostomy, gastroparesis 171
genes
    bladder problems 194
    diabetic neuropathy 148
    monogenic forms 57
    type 1 diabetes 35
    type 2 diabetes 42
Genetic and Rare Diseases Information Center
    (GARD)
    publications
        acanthosis nigricans (AN) 191n
        necrobiosis lipoidica 191n
genetic testing, monogenic diabetes
GES *see* gastric electrical stimulation
gestational diabetes
    carbohydrate counting 271
    described 10
    diabetic eye disease 156
    overview 51–5
    prediabetes 29
    type 2 diabetes 41
    urine test 98
"Gestational Diabetes and Pregnancy" (CDC) 51n
gingivitis
    oral health 135
    plaque 176
glaucoma, vision 136
glucagon
    emergency 231
    hypoglycemia 120
    pediatric patients 108
    type 1 diabetes 33
"Glucose in Urine Test" (NIH) 97n
glucose meters
    carbohydrate counting 271
    described 91
    type 1 diabetes 38
glucose tablets
    backpack checklist 212
    hypoglycemia 120
    traveling 224
gum disease
    blood glucose control 211
    diabetes 44

gum disease, *continued*
    glucose 175
    hyperglycemia 122
    oral health 135
gums *see* oral health

H

hammertoes, right type of shoes 186
HDL *see* high-density lipoprotein
healthcare team
    foot check 187
    hypoglycemia 220
    meal plan 262
    pregnancy concerns 197
    sexual and bladder problems 193
    weight-loss plan 261
healthy diet
    diabetes treatment and management 240
    type 2 diabetes 277
healthy eating
    quick tips 249
    see also diet and nutrition
"Healthy Eating for Diabetics" (VA) 249n
"Healthy Weight" (CDC) 285n
heart attack
    blood pressure 78
    carbohydrate counting 267
    family history 141
    plaque 17
    smoking 180
heart disease
    diabetes 131
    family history 141
    metabolic syndrome 17
    omega-3 fatty acid supplements 275
    risk 20
    statins 23
hematocrit, blood glucose monitoring 91
hemoglobin A1C test (HbA1c test), described 48
high blood glucose *see* hyperglycemia
high blood pressure *see* hypertension
high-density lipoprotein (HDL)
    abnormal cholesterol levels 140
    metabolic risk factors 22
Hispanics
    diabetic eye disease 155
    kidney disease 162
    type 1 and type 2 diabetes 14

HIV *see* human immunodeficiency viruses
hormone
    fighting sickness 227
    insulin 27
    menstrual cycle 54
"How to Help Students Implement Effective Diabetes Management" (NIDDK) 121n
human immunodeficiency viruses (HIV), insulin resistance 29
hybrid closed-loop system, artificial pancreas system 38
hyperglycemia (high blood glucose)
    blood sugar level 85
    diabetes management 211
    diabetic ketoacidosis (DKA) 101
    driving 220
    gastroparesis 170
    genetic testing 59
    management 121
hypertension (high blood pressure)
    gestational diabetes 106
    heart disease 131
    maturity-onset diabetes of the young (MODY) 59
    metabolic syndrome 18
    pregnancy 52
hypoglycemia (low blood glucose)
    autonomic neuropathy 148
    blood glucose control 211
    blood sugar level 85
    diabetes medicines 108
    management 115
    symptoms 244
hypoglycemia unawareness
    continuous glucose monitoring (CGM) 95
    described 118
hypothyroidism, gastroparesis 168

I

"Importance of Wearing Medical Alert Bracelets and Necklaces" (Omnigraphics) 215n
Indiana University Diabetes Translational Research Program, contact 302
ingrown toenails, foot problem 184
injection aids, insulin intake devices 113
injection ports, insulin intake devices 112
insulin
    delivery devices 111

insulin, *continued*
    described 27
    diabetes 3
    gestational diabetes 51
    ketones 102
    neonatal diabetes mellitus (NDM) 58
    prediabetes 31
    type 1 diabetes 13
    type 2 diabetes 41
"Insulin" (FDA) 111n
insulin jet injectors, insulin delivery devices 113
"Insulin, Medicines, and Other Diabetes Treatments"
    (NIDDK) 105n
insulin pens, insulin delivery devices 111
insulin pumps, insulin delivery devices 49
insulin resistance
    described 27
    excess weight 30
    metabolic syndrome risk 18
    vitamin D 276
"Insulin Resistance and Prediabetes" (NIDDK) 27n
intrauterine devices (IUDs), birth control 54
IUDs *see* intrauterine devices

J

jejunostomy, gastroparesis 171
jejunum, gastroparesis 171
jet injectors, insulin delivery devices 113
Johns Hopkins Diabetes Center, contact 302
Joslin Diabetes and Endocrinology Research Center
    (DERC), contact 296
Joslin Diabetes Center, contact 302
Juvenile Diabetes Research Foundation (JDRF),
    contact 307

K

ketones
    diabetic ketoacidosis 122
    insulin delivery devices 112
    neonatal diabetes mellitus (NDM) 58
    physical activity and diabetes 283
    urine test 101
    see also diabetic ketoacidosis
"Ketones in Urine" (NIH) 101n
kidney disease
    carbohydrate counting 267

kidney disease, *continued*
    dietary supplements 277
    overview 161–5
    smoking and diabetes 239
    tooth and gum problems **176**
    weight-loss surgery 290
    see also chronic kidney disease
kidney failure, diabetic kidney disease 162
kidneys
    A1C test 78
    diabetes-related health concerns 132
    hyperglycemia treatment 122
    metabolic syndrome 24
    monogenic diabetes 59
    pregnancy 233
"Know Your Blood Sugar Numbers: Use Them to
    Manage Your Diabetes" (NIDDK) 83n

L

laser surgery, vision 136
Latinx
    diabetes risk 11
    diabetic eye disease 155
    type 2 diabetes 41
LDL *see* low-density lipoprotein
lifestyle
    carbohydrate counting 271
    diabetes medicines **107**
    diabetes treatment fraud 125
    diabetic kidney disease 163
    insulin resistance 32
    metabolic syndrome 20
    monogenic diabetes 62
    prediabetes 9
    type 2 diabetes 42
liver
    diabetes medicines 107
    heart disease 140
    herbal supplements 274
    insulin 27
    metabolic syndrome 19
low blood glucose *see* hypoglycemia
"Low Blood Glucose (Hypoglycemia)"
    (NIDDK) 115n
low-density lipoprotein (LDL)
    cholesterol 78
    heart attack 142
    heart disease risk 20

low-density lipoprotein (LDL), *continued*
    medical alert bracelet 215
    physical activity and diabetes 280
lung disease, heart disease 140

M

macula
    diabetic eye disease 153
    dietary supplements 273
    unapproved diabetes drugs 126
macular edema
    diabetic eye disease 153
    dietary supplements 273
malnutrition, gastroparesis 169
"Managing Diabetes in the Heat" (CDC) 235n
Massachusetts General Hospital (MGH) Diabetes
    Clinical Research Center, contact 299
maturity-onset diabetes of the young (MODY),
    monogenic diabetes 57
meal plan *see also* spa menu
mealtime
    healthy eating 249
    type 1 diabetes 38
medical devices, type 2 diabetes 110
medical emergency
    diabetic eye disease **156**
    ketones 101
    managing diabetes 235
    managing hyperglycemia 121
    medical alert bracelets 215
medications
    acanthosis nigricans (AN) 192
    blood glucose control 211
    diabetes care team **70**
    hyperglycemia 121
    low blood sugar 53
    metabolic syndrome 23
    obesity 141
    overview 105–10
    smoking **240**
    weight-loss surgery 290
meglitinide, hypoglycemia 117
menstrual cycle, gestational diabetes 54
mental health
    diabetes care team 71
    health concerns 136
    overview 203–6
metabolic factors, diabetic neuropathy **149**

metabolic syndrome
    heart disease 132
    overview 17–25
    vitamins 276
"Metabolic Syndrome" (NHLBI) 17n
metformin
    gestational diabetes 106
    insulin resistance 32
metoclopramide, medicines 170
Michigan Diabetes Research Center (MDRC),
    contact 299
microalbumin, kidney disease 133
miglitol, hypoglycemia 120
MiniMed Paradigm REAL-Time System, artificial
    pancreas 114
"Monogenic Diabetes (Neonatal Diabetes Mellitus
    and MODY)" (NIDDK) 57n
multivitamin, eating habits 169
mutation, monogenic diabetes 57

N

National Center for Complementary and Integrative
    Health (NCCIH)
        contact 303
        publication
            diabetes and dietary supplements 273n
National Certification Board For Diabetes Educators
    (NCBDE), contact 307
National Diabetes Education Program (NDEP),
    contact 295
National Diabetes Information Clearinghouse
    (NDIC), contact 295
National Digestive Diseases Information
    Clearinghouse (NDDIC), contact 295
National Eye Institute (NEI), contact 303
National Glycohemoglobin Standardization Program
    (NGSP), contact 307
National Heart, Lung, and Blood Institute
    (NHLBI)
        contact 304
        publication
            metabolic syndrome 17n
National Highway Traffic Safety Administration
    (NHTSA)
        publication
            diabetes and driving 219n
National Institute of Arthritis and Musculoskeletal
    and Skin Diseases (NIAMS), contact 298, 304

National Institute of Dental and Craniofacial Research (NIDCR), contact 299, 304

National Institute of Diabetes and Digestive and Kidney Diseases (NIDDK)
  contact 296
  publications
    alternative devices for taking insulin 111n
    blood sugar numbers 83n
    carbohydrate counting and diabetes 265n
    continuous glucose monitoring (CGM) 89n
    diabetes 3n
    diabetes and foot problems 183n
    diabetes care during sick days and special times 227n
    diabetes diet, eating, and physical activity 259n
    diabetes, gum disease, and other dental problems 175n
    diabetes, heart disease, and stroke 139n
    diabetes management at school 211n
    diabetes, sexual, and bladder problems 193n
    diabetic eye disease 153n
    diabetic kidney disease 161n
    diabetic neuropathy 147n
    foot and skin problems caused by diabetes 183n
    gastroparesis 167n
    insulin, medicines, and other diabetes treatments 105n
    insulin resistance and prediabetes 27n
    low blood glucose (hypoglycemia) 115n
    managing diabetes 75n
    managing hyperglycemia 121n
    monogenic forms of diabetes 57n
    type 1 diabetes 33n
    type 2 diabetes 41n

National Institute on Aging (NIA), contact 304

National Institutes of Health (NIH)
  publications
    diabetes in children and teens 13n
    early weight-loss surgery and improvement in type 2 diabetes, blood pressure outcomes 289n
    glucose in urine test 97n
    ketones in urine 101n

National Institutes of Health Osteoporosis and Related Bone Diseases—National Resource Center (NIH ORBD—NRC), contact 298

National Kidney and Urologic Diseases Information Clearinghouse (NKUDIC), contact 296

National Kidney Disease Education Program (NKDEP), contact 296

National Kidney Foundation (NKF), contact 307

Native Hawaiians
  family history **43**
  gestational diabetes 11
  prediabetes 29

NDEP see National Diabetes Education Program

NDIC see National Diabetes Information Clearinghouse

necrobiosis lipoidica, described 192

"Necrobiosis Lipoidica" (GARD) 191n

NEI see National Eye Institute

The Nemours Foundation/KidsHealth®, contact 303

neonatal diabetes mellitus (NDM), monogenic forms of diabetes 57

nerve damage
  diabetes care team 69
  diabetic neuropathy 150
  dietary supplements 273
  gastroparesis 172
  gestational diabetes 51
  mental health 203
  overview 133–6
  pregnancy 233
  skin 189
  type 1 diabetes 38

nervous system
  gastroparesis 168
  nerve damage 133
  selenium 276

neurovascular factors, diabetic neuropathy **149**

NHTSA see National Highway Traffic Safety Administration

NIDDK see National Institute of Diabetes and Digestive and Kidney Diseases

NIH see National Institutes of Health

non-starchy vegetables
  healthy eating 249
  meal plan methods 262

nonproliferative diabetic retinopathy, diabetic eye disease 154

nutrition
  diabetes care team 72
  gastroparesis 171
  healthy eating 251
  healthy weight 285

Nutrition Facts label
  carbohydrates 251
  metabolic syndrome **24**
  traveling 224

O

obesity
    acanthosis nigricans (AN) 191
    children and adolescents 13
    excess weight 30
    heart disease 132
    monogenic diabetes 59
    weight-loss planning 261
    weight-loss surgery 289
Office of Minority Health Resource Center
    (OMHRC), contact 302, 305
OGTT *see* oral glucose tolerance test
omega-3 fatty acids, dietary supplements 275
OMHRC *see* Office of Minority Health Reference
    Center
Omnigraphics
    publications
        double diabetes 47n
        medical alert bracelets and necklaces 215n
oral burning, tabulated *178*
oral glucose tolerance test (OGTT)
    double diabetes 49
    insulin resistance 31
oral health, described 135
oral rehydration solutions, gastroparesis 169
overweight
    bladder problems 194
    diabetes myths **65**
    diabetic kidney disease 162
    diabetic neuropathy 148
    heart disease 132
    insulin resistance 28
    meal plans and diabetes 261
    metabolic syndrome 18
    monogenic forms of diabetes 59
    prediabetes 10
    smoking and diabetes 240
    type 2 diabetes 4
    weight and exercise 286
    weight-loss surgery **291**

P

Pacific Islanders
    diabetic eye disease 155
    genes and family history **43**
    prediabetes 10
PAD *see* peripheral artery disease

painful sex, sexual problems 196
pancreas
    carbohydrate counting 266
    diabetes 3
    insulin 27
    monogenic diabetes 57
    smoking and diabetes 239
    type 2 diabetes 41
pancreatitis, diabetes medicines 109
panretinal photocoagulation (PRP), diabetic eye
    disease 158
parenteral nutrition, gastroparesis 171
PCOS *see* polycystic ovary syndrome
Pedorthic Footcare Association (PFA), contact 308
penile curvature, sexual problems 195
periodontitis, tooth and gum problems 176
peripheral artery disease (PAD), foot problems 188
peripheral neuropathy
    diabetic neuropathy 147
    nerve damage 133
    smoking and diabetes 240
Peyronie disease, sexual problems 195
photocoagulation, diabetic eye disease 157
physical activity
    continuous glucose monitoring (CGM) 94
    diabetes care team **72**
    diabetes management 211
    diabetes medicines 105
    diabetes myths 64
    diabetes-related health concerns 132
    diabetic kidney disease 163
    dietary supplements **276**
    gestational diabetes **52**
    healthy eating for diabetics **250**
    hyperglycemia 121
    insulin resistance 30
    meal plans and diabetes 261
    metabolic syndrome 18
    prediabetes 9
    sexual or bladder problems 199
    smoking and diabetes 240
    type 1 diabetes 36
    type 2 diabetes 44
    weight and exercise 286
    see also exercises
plaque
    metabolic syndrome 17
    penile curvature 195
    tooth and gum problems 175

plate method
    described 262
    healthy eating 249
podiatrist
    diabetes care team 70
    foot problems 134
polycystic ovary syndrome (PCOS)
    gestational diabetes 11
    insulin resistance 29
    sexual problems 197
pramlintide, type 1 diabetes 36
pregnancy
    carbohydrate counting 271
    diabetes medicines 106
    diabetes myths 63
    diabetic eye disease 155
    gestational diabetes 4, **52**
    glucose in urine test 98
    insulin resistance and prediabetes 31
    risk for diabetes 10
    sexual and bladder problems 197
    type 2 diabetes 43
Prevent Blindness, contact 297
"Prevent Complications" (CDC) 131n
"Prevent Diabetes Problems: Keep Your Feet and Skin
    Healthy" (NIDDK) 183n
proliferative diabetic retinopathy, vitrectomy 158
protein
    carbohydrate counting 265
    diabetes myths 64
    double diabetes 49
    healthy eating 249
    healthy food for diabetics 310
    kidney disease 133
    meal plans and diabetes 259
    monogenic diabetes 57
proximal neuropathy, diabetic neuropathy 148
puberty, diabetes management 211

Q

QOL *see* quality of life
quality of life (QOL), gastroparesis 168

R

ranibizumab, diabetic eye disease 157

"Rates of New Diagnosed Cases of Type 1 and Type 2
    Diabetes on the Rise among Children, Teens"
    (NIH) 13n
recipes, overview 309–24
red meat, metabolic syndrome **24**
retinopathy
    insulin resistance 30
    smoking and diabetes 240
risk factors
    diabetes care team 70
    diabetic neuropathy **149**
    insulin resistance 28
    metabolic syndrome 17
    monogenic diabetes 57
    type 1 diabetes 9
    type 2 diabetes 44

S

safety considerations
    automobile driving 222
    dietary supplements 274
    insulin delivery devices 113
salt
    diabetes meal plan 79
    foods and drinks to limit **252**
    healthy lifestyle 164
    heart disease 131
saturated fat
    foods and drinks to limit **260**
    healthy food for diabetics 309
    Nutrition Facts label 256
scatter laser treatment, diabetic eye disease 158
school nurses
    diabetes management at school 212
    healthcare team 71
school settings
    diabetes management 211
    hyperglycemia **123**
    sick days 229
scleroderma, gastroparesis 168
seizure
    driving and diabetes 219
    gestational diabetes 52
    hypoglycemia 116
severe headache, stroke 145
severe hypoglycemia, type 1 diabetes 36
sexual problems, overview 193–9
sexually transmitted diseases (STDs), sexual and
    bladder problems of diabetes 197

side effects
    diabetes, heart disease, and stroke 143
    diabetes management 80
    diabetes medicines 108
    dietary supplements 274
    hypoglycemia 117
    sexual and bladder problems 195
"6 Things to Know about Type 2 Diabetes and
    Dietary Supplements" (NCCIH) 273n
skim milk, diabetes management 79
skin
    acanthosis nigricans (AN) 191
    diabetes effects 183
    insulin delivery devices 111
    insulin resistance and prediabetes 30
skin tags, insulin resistance and prediabetes 30
smoking
    diabetes, heart disease, and stroke 140
    diabetes-related health concerns 132
    diabetic eye disease 153
    diabetic neuropathy 148
    foot and skin problems 187
    healthy lifestyle habits 164
    overview 239–41
    sexual and bladder problems 199
    tooth and gum problems 180
    type 2 diabetes 42
"Smoking and Diabetes" (CDC) 239n
sodium
    healthy food for diabetics 309
    healthy lifestyle habits 164
    meal plans 260
    Nutrition Facts label 256
sores
    diabetes management 80
    diabetic neuropathy 150
    foot problems 134
    necrobiosis lipoidica 192
    type 2 diabetes 42
spa menu, traveling with diabetes 225
starches
    carbohydrate counting 266
    diabetes myths 64
    healthy eating for diabetics 249
    healthy food choices 255
    meal plans and diabetes 262
    tooth and gum problems 175
statistics
    diabetes incidence and prevalence 6
    race, ethnicity, and education 7

"Stay Healthy" (CDC) 285n
STDs see sexually transmitted diseases
stress
    coping 69, 207
    diabetes, heart disease, and stroke 143
    diabetes management 79
    diabetic kidney disease 164
    healthy weight 287
    mental health and diabetes 137, 204
    overview 207–9
stress incontinence, sexual and bladder problems of
    diabetes 198
stroke
    carbohydrate counting 267
    diabetes management at school 211
    managing diabetes in the heat 235
    metabolic syndrome 23
    overview 139–45
    smoking 180
sugar
    blood sugar 83
    carbohydrate counting 265
    diabetes 3
    diabetes and mental health 204
    diabetes management 78
    diabetes medicines 108
    diabetes-related health concerns 135
    dietary supplements 275
    double diabetes 49
    family health history and diabetes 11
    gestational diabetes 53
    healthy eating for diabetics 251, 309
    hypoglycemia 115
    making healthy food choices 255
    managing diabetes in the heat 236
    meal plans 261
    metabolic syndrome 18
    physical activity and diabetes 283
    tooth and gum problems 175
    traveling with diabetes 225
sugar diabetes see diabetes mellitus
sugar substitutes, healthy eating for diabetics 251
sulfonylureas
    diabetes medicines 109
    hypoglycemia 117
    monogenic forms of diabetes 59
surgery
    diabetic eye disease 158
    weight loss 289

sweat glands
    diabetic neuropathy 148
    managing diabetes in the heat 235
sweating
    diabetes and mental health 204
    diabetes, heart disease, and stroke 144
    foot and skin problems 189
    hypoglycemia 117
symlin (pramlintide), type 1 diabetes 36
syndrome X *see* metabolic syndrome
syringes
    coping with diabetes distress 208
    emergency or a natural disaster happens 231
    insulin delivery devices 113

T

"Take Care of Your Diabetes during Sick Days and
    Special Times" (NIDDK) 227n
tartar, tooth and gum problems 176
"Team Care Approach for Diabetes Management"
    (CDC) 69n
TEDDY study, diabetes in children and
    adolescents 16
teeth *see* oral health
"10 Tips for Coping with Diabetes Distress" (CDC) 207n
test strips
    blood glucose monitoring 90
    coping with diabetes distress 208
    hyperglycemia 122
    ketones in urine test 103
    managing diabetes in the heat 237
    traveling with diabetes 224
testosterone, sexual problems 195
tests
    double diabetes 48
    metabolic syndrome 21
tobacco use
    diabetes healthcare team 69
    diabetes, heart disease, and stroke 142
    diabetes medicines 110
    smoking and diabetes **240**
TODAY (Treatment Options for Type 1 Diabetes in
    Adolescents and Youth) study, diabetes in children
    and adolescents 16
trans fat
    diabetes management 79
    foods and drinks to limit 260
    healthy food for diabetics 309
    Nutrition Facts label 256

transplantation
    diabetes treatment **107**
    type 1 diabetes 38
transportation security administration (TSA),
    traveling with diabetes 224
travel considerations, overview 223–5
"Treatment for Gastroparesis" (NIDDK) 167n
"Trends in Diabetic Ketoacidosis Hospitalizations
    and In-Hospital Mortality—United States,
    2000–2014" (CDC) 101n
triglyceride
    diabetes, heart disease, and stroke 141
    diabetes-related health concerns 132
    diabetic neuropathy 148
    metabolic syndrome 17
TSA *see* transportation security administration
"21 Tips for Traveling with Diabetes" (CDC) 223n
type 1 diabetes
    diabetes in children and adolescents 15
    diabetes medicines 105
    diabetes statistics 5
    diabetic kidney disease 163
    double diabetes 47
    hypoglycemia 116
    monogenic forms of diabetes 58
    overview 33–9
"Type 1 Diabetes" (NIDDK) 33n
type 2 diabetes
    diabetes in children and adolescents 14
    diabetes medicines 105
    diabetes-related health concerns 132
    diabetes statistics 4
    dietary supplements 276
    double diabetes 47
    gestational diabetes **52**
    healthy weight 286
    insulin resistance and prediabetes 31
    metabolic syndrome 22
    monogenic forms of diabetes 59
    overview 41–5
    smoking and diabetes 240
    weight-loss surgery 289
"Type 2 Diabetes" (NIDDK) 41n

U

ulcers
    hot spot 184
    nerve damage 185
    peripheral neuropathy 150
    smoking 140, 240

The University of Chicago Diabetes Research and
   Training Center (DRTC), contact 300
University of Colorado Diabetes and Endocrinology
   Research Center (DERC), contact 297
University of Washington Diabetes Research Center
   (DRC), contact 300
urinary frequency, diabetes 198
urinary incontinence, bladder problem 197
urinary tract, neuropathy 193
urinary tract infections (UTI)
      bladder infections 198
      diabetes complications 135
      women's diabetes complications 53
urine test
      bladder problems 198
      diabetic kidney disease 162
      glucose, overview 97–9
      ketones, overview 101–4
      women's sexual problems 196
Urology Care Foundation, contact 301, 308
U.S. Department of Veterans Affairs (VA)
      publication
            diabetes and healthy eating 249n
U.S. Food and Drug Administration (FDA)
      publications
            blood glucose monitoring devices 89n
            diabetes medicines 105n
            diabetes treatment fraud 125n
            insulin 111n

V

VA *see* U.S. Department of Veterans Affairs
vagus nerve, gastroparesis 168
Vanderbilt Diabetes Research and Training Center
   (DRTC), contact 300
vegetables
      carbohydrate counting 265
      diabetes 50, 269
      healthy eating 253, 310
      plate method 249, 262
venting gastrostomy, described 171
Victoza (liraglutide), pediatric patients 108–9
visceral fat, insulin resistance 30
vision
      diabetes complications 136
      diabetic retinopathy 156
vision loss
      diabetes 159
      diabetic eye disease 153

vision problems
      diabetes complications 42, 220, 245
      diabetic eye disease 154
      double diabetes 48
      hyperglycemia 85
      metabolic syndrome 19
      mild-to-moderate hypoglycemia 116
      type 1 diabetes 34
      see also eyes; retinopathy
vitrectomy, described 158
vitreous gel, diabetic eye disease 158

W

Washington University School of Medicine
   (WUSM) Diabetes Research Center (DRC),
   contact 300
Weight-Control Information Network (WIN),
   contact 296
weight management, bariatric surgery 290
"What are the Causes of Sinus Infections?"
   (CDC) 9n
"What Is Diabetes?" (NIDDK) 3n
"What Is Diabetic Neuropathy?"
   (NIDDK) 147n
"What Is Effective Diabetes Management at School?"
   (NIDDK) 211n
whole grains
      carbohydrate counting 263, 265
      diabetes 259
      healthy choices 253, 310
WIN *see* Weight-Control Information Network
WUSM *see* Washington University School of
   Medicine

X

X-ray machine, insulin pump 224, 230
xerostomia, mouth problem *178*

Y

Yale Diabetes Research Center (DRC), contact 300
yoga, stress management 143, 205

Z

zucchini, non-starchy vegetables 250, 266